MW01626328

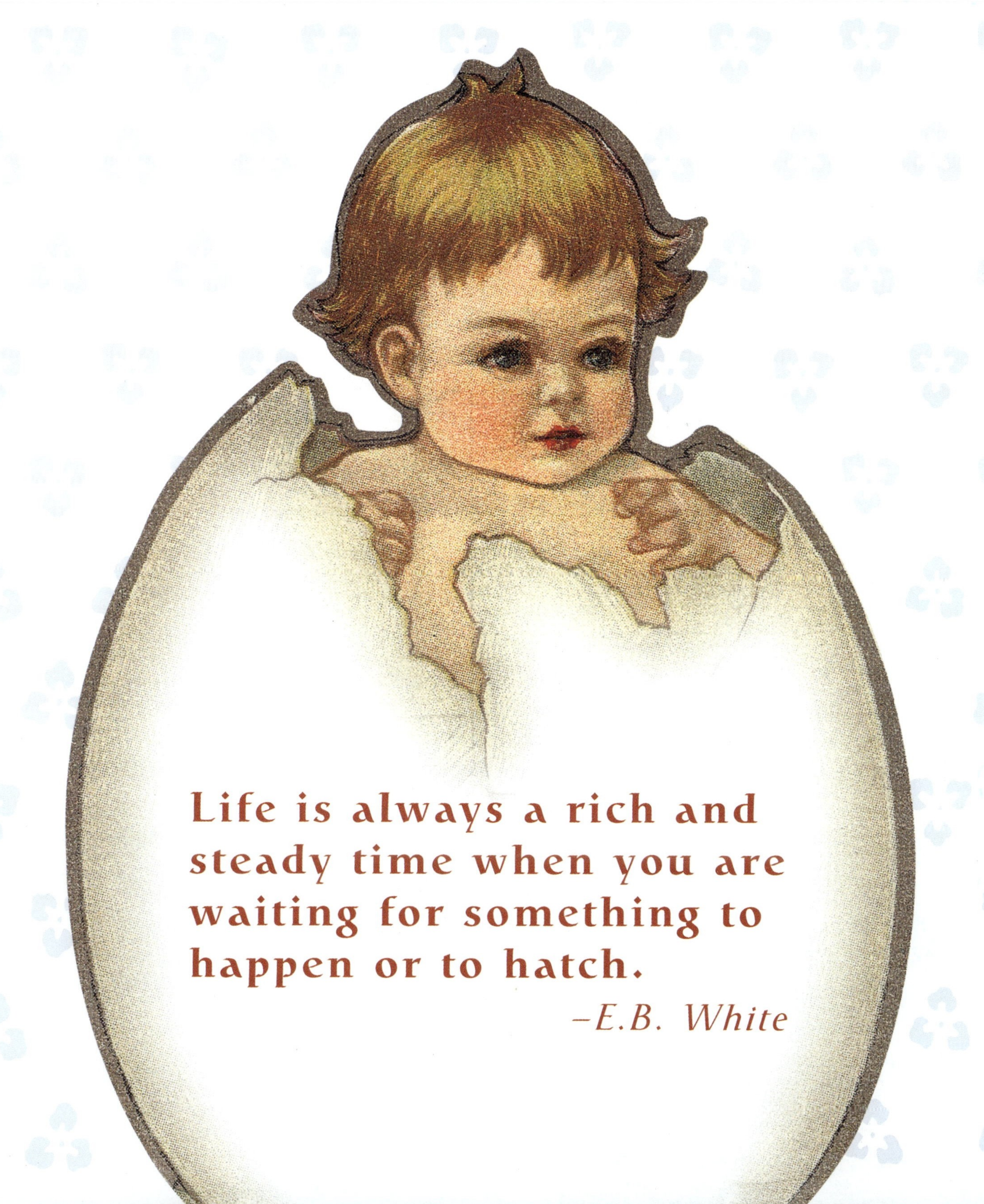

Life is always a rich and steady time when you are waiting for something to happen or to hatch.

–*E.B. White*

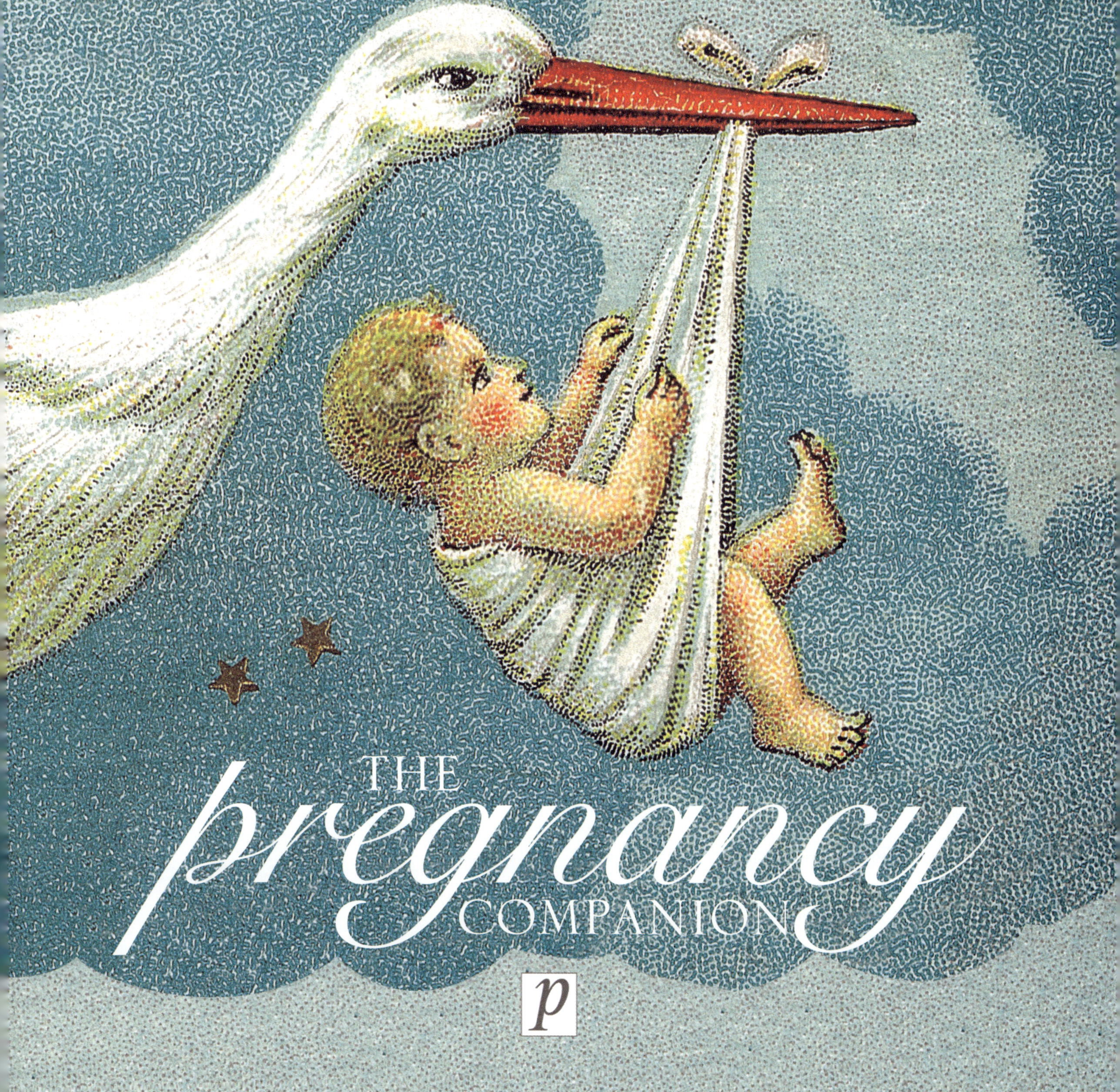
THE
pregnancy
COMPANION
p

This is a Parragon Publishing Book
This edition published in 2006

Parragon Publishing
Queen Street House
4 Queen Street
Bath BA1 1HE, UK

Designer: Jon Glick
Editorial and Research Assistants: Lawrence Chesler, Rachel Hertz, Nicholas Liu, Miki Raver

Home Remedies, Old Wives Tales, & Traditions
written by Svea Vocke
Recipes by Sara Baysinger
Activities by Marsha Heckman

Copyright © 2006 Welcome Enterprises, Inc.

All rights reserved. No part of this book may be reproduced or utilized in any form or by any means, electronic or mechanical, including photocopying, recording, or by any information storage or retrieval system, without permission in writing from the copyright holders.

Printed in Singapore
10 9 8 7 6 5 4 3 2 1

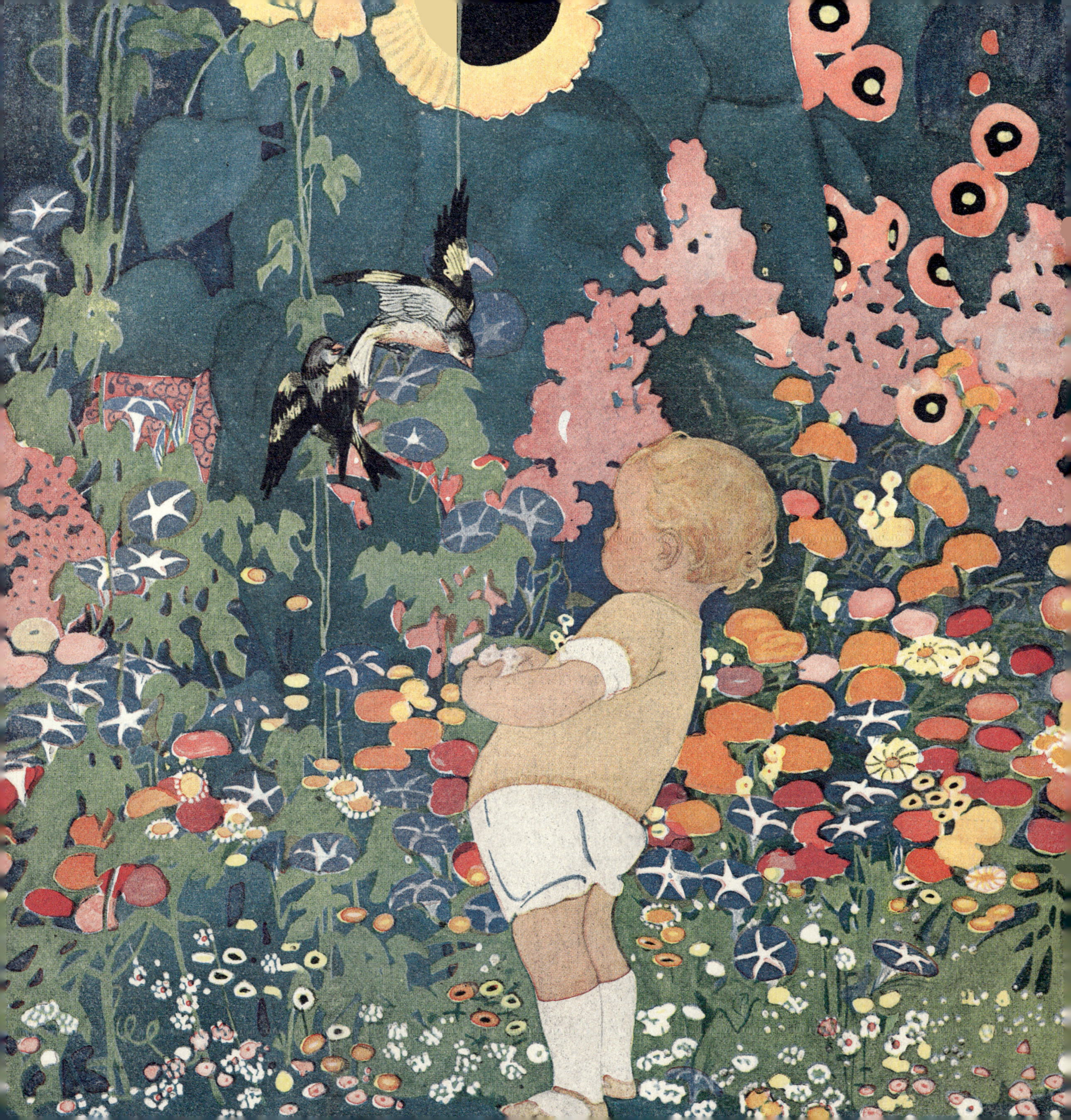

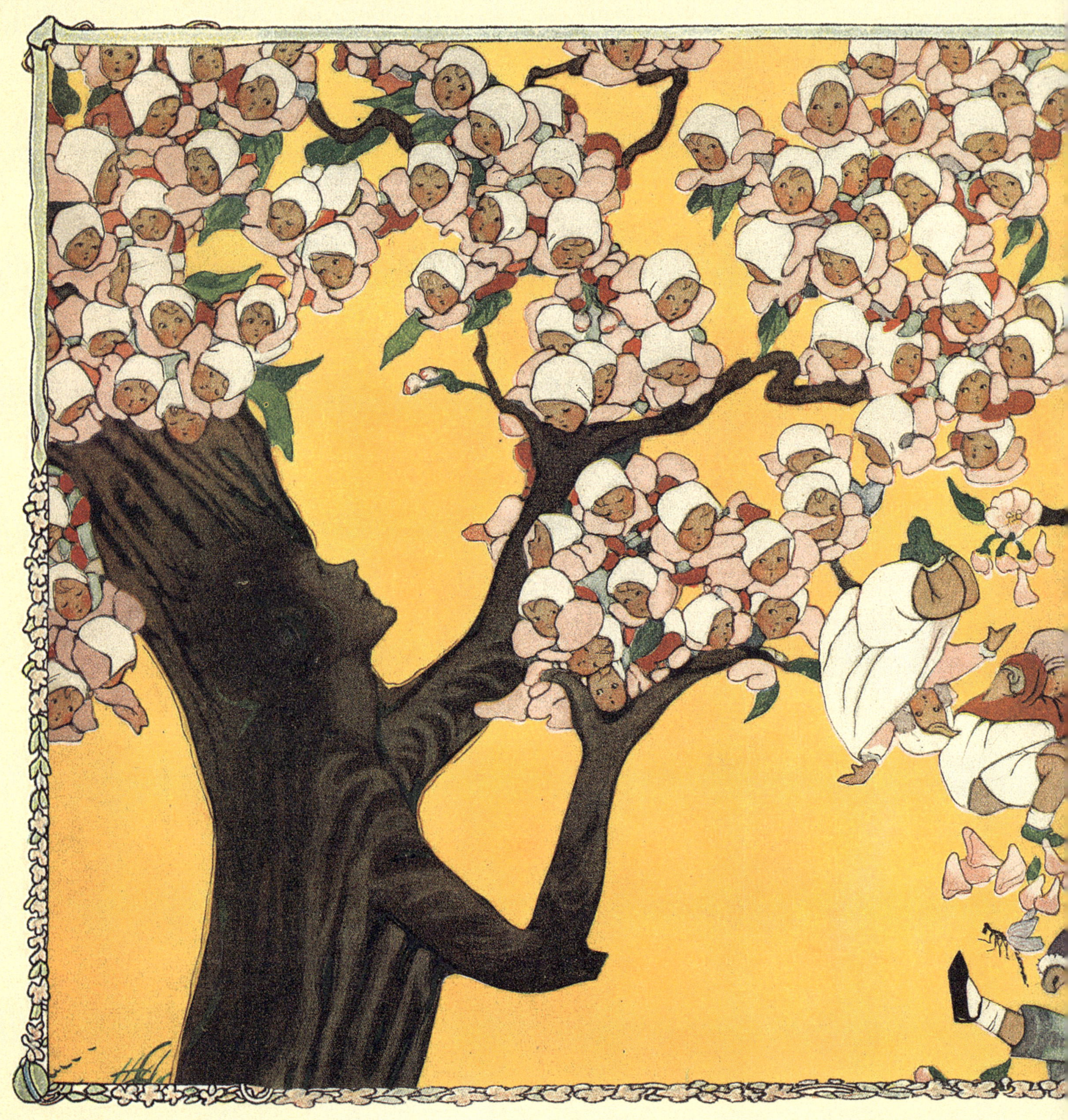

CONTENTS

OLD WIVES' TALES

TRADITIONS & INSPIRATION

FACTS & FUN

HOME REMEDIES

ACTIVITIES

RECIPES

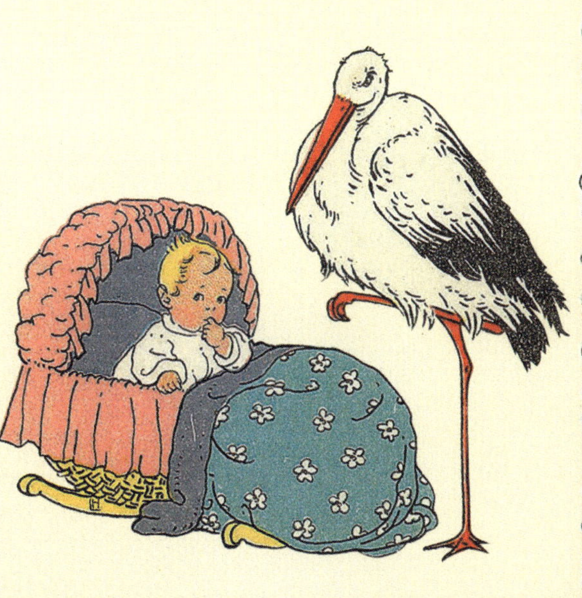

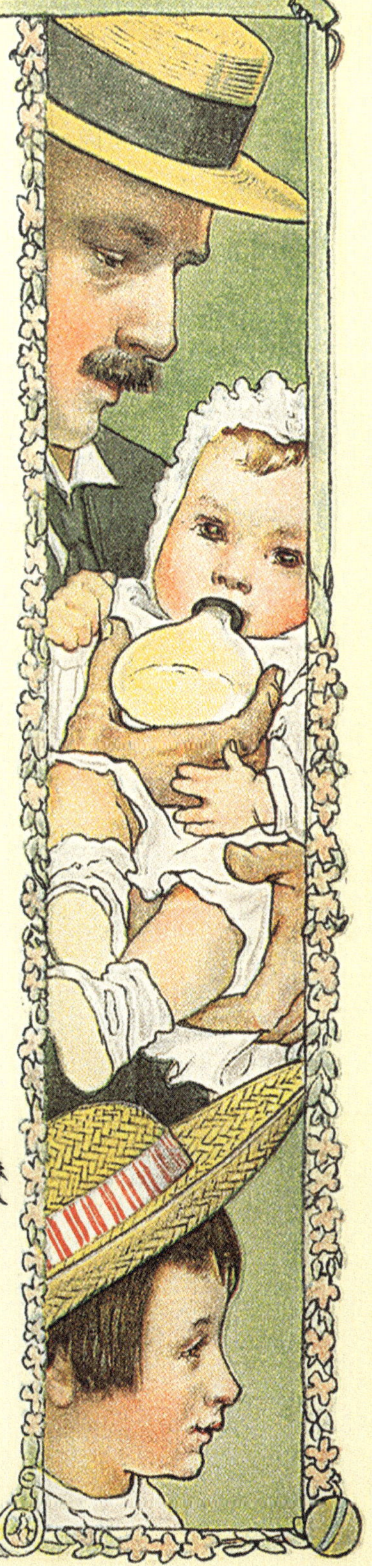

Making the decision to have
a child—it's momentous.
It is to decide forever to
have your heart go walking
around outside your body.

—Elizabeth Stone

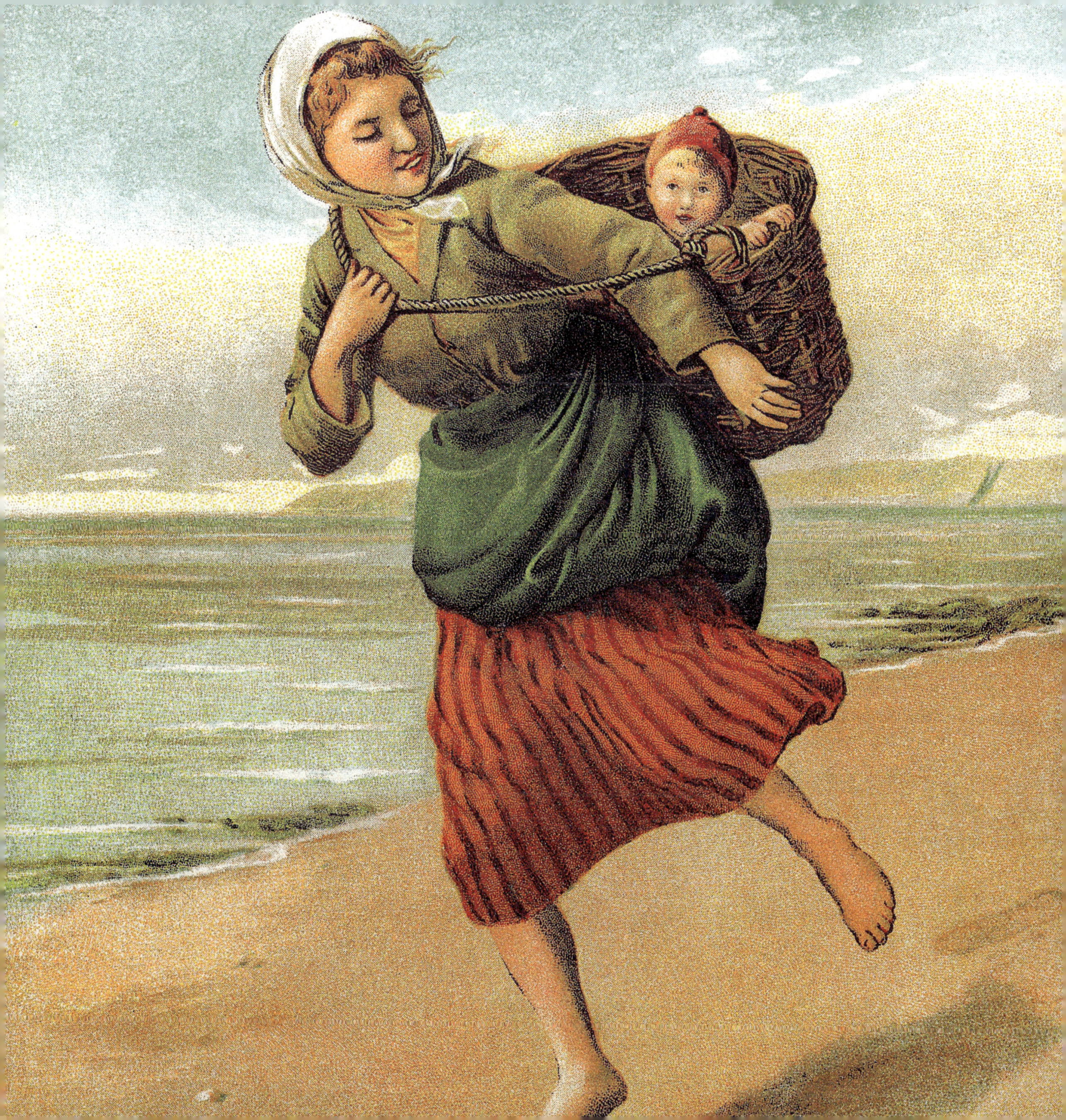

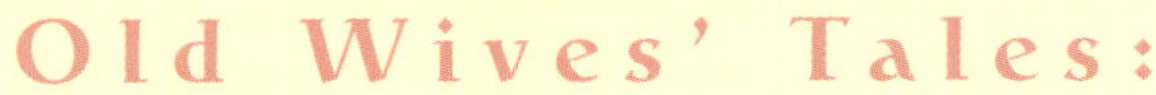

Old Wives' Tales:

Baby on the Way

Thinking back, what made you first think you were pregnant? Did you have trouble concentrating? Were you unusually tired? Emotional? Nauseated? "Late"? Before the days of fertility drugs and pregnancy tests, women had little more than their hopes and intuition to work with. Or did they? Throughout history, people have tried to encourage and predict conception. Read on and judge some of the more old-fashioned methods for yourself.

The Celtic Druids gathered acorns and carried pine cones to promote fertility. In some parts of ancient England, Germany, and Scandinavia where oak trees were said to be favored by the Norse god Thor, acorns also were considered to be totems of sexual power. The Romans and Greeks carried flowers and herbs to protect against illness and encourage fertility. Other traditional fertility talismans include horseshoes and the more well-known mistletoe.

Wedding ceremonies have long been rich with fertility rites. Wedding cakes supposedly began as the sweet cakes of Roman times which were

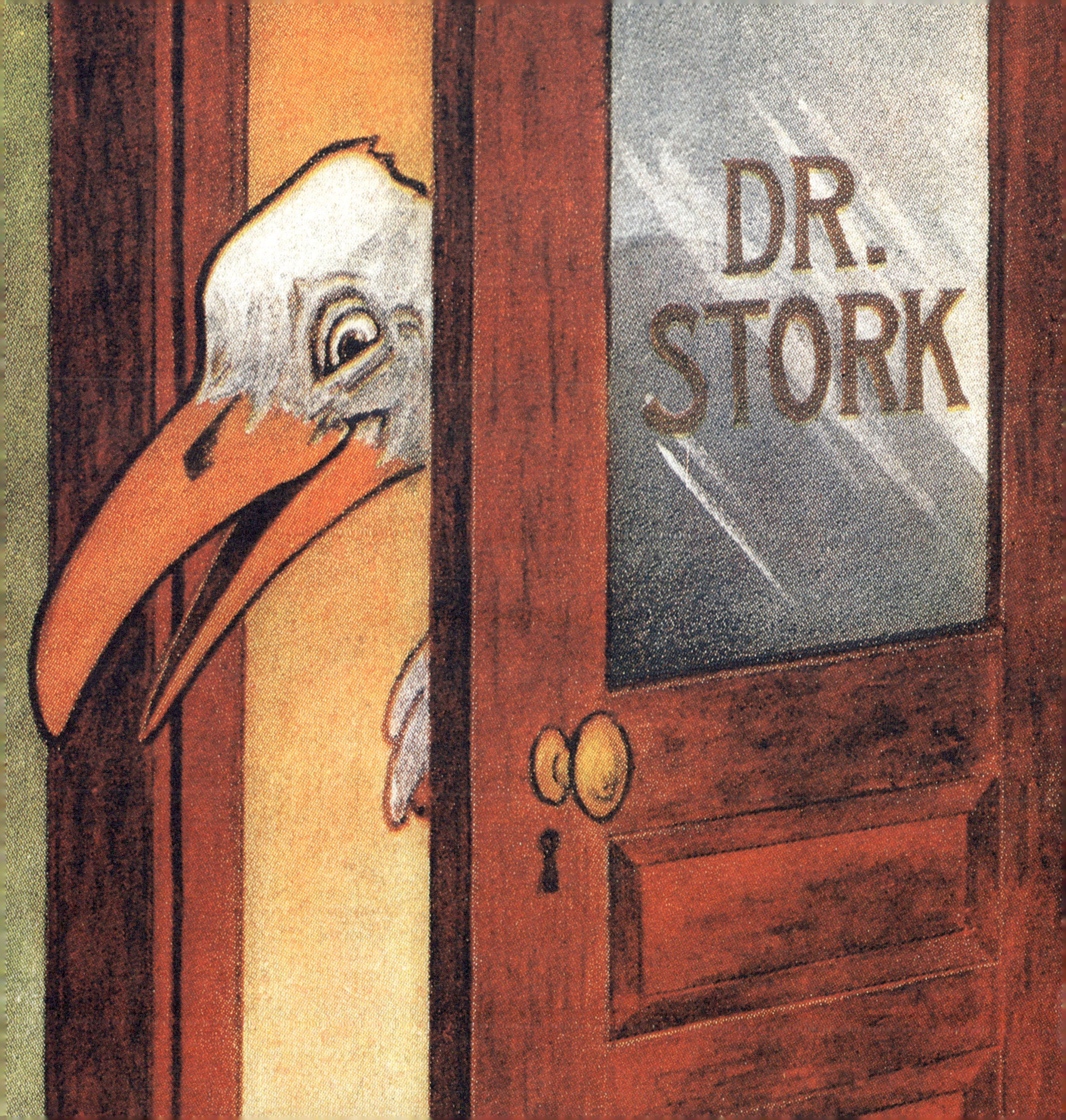
DR.
STORK

thought to bring fertility, happiness, and abundance. Ever wonder why you throw rice at a new bride and groom? Some say the tradition began as guests throwing bits of the wedding cake, or by crumbling bread over the couple's heads, or by showering the couple with wheat or corn. But whatever its origin, the throwing of grain—a symbol of bountiful harvests—is clearly meant to encourage fertility. Even sprays of baby's breath, now a common element of the bridal bouquet, began as fertility symbols.

Newlyweds have always been swamped with baby expectations. An American folktale says that stuffing garlic in the keyhole of your honeymoon-suite door ensures a quick pregnancy. Another eastern European fertility custom is said to be the origin of the "cat's cradle." Cats were often considered symbols of fertility, and after a wedding, a cat was put in a cradle and taken to the newlyweds' house. For a sure-fire, speedy conception, the cat was then rocked in the couple's presence.

Many traditions and superstitions surround the prediction of childbirth as well. Jewish scholars wrote that if a man dreamed of a vineyard, of sleeping under trees, or of carrying a bird in his bosom it foretold of future children. Others believe that baby dreams mean a child will be born into your family. Fish dreams suggest someone you know is pregnant.

If you have trouble sleeping, take a peek out your window. A bright star predicts that someone will soon give birth. If your right eye starts to twitch, that's the sign of an imminent birth in your family. In the morning, you might look for a rainbow. On the Orkney Islands (off Scotland), a bright rainbow preceded the birth of a boy. If you're distracted by a rabbit running across your yard, know that the bounding bunny means that this year will be a good time to have children. And if you're getting dressed and realize you've lost a pair of earrings, a Guatemalan folktale asserts you will surely become pregnant within six short months.

Of course, many beliefs center on babies themselves. If a married woman is the first to see a newborn, she will be the next to have a baby. A woman who holds an infant on her first visit to a new mother will soon be a mother too. Find a baby's pacifier and your family can expect a baby soon. And a wives' tale version of Murphy's Law warns that giving away outgrown baby clothes will mean you'll inevitably need them again soon.

Our last tale sounds like an assertion any astute, overprotective mother might rally behind. Rumor has it that a woman who lays her hat or coat on an unfamiliar bed will soon become pregnant. Hmmm...wonder where the Old Wives got that idea?

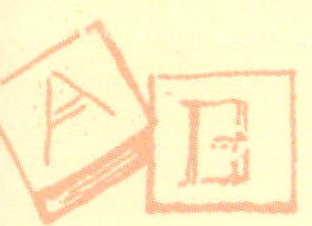

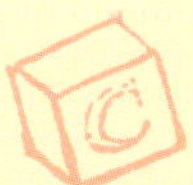

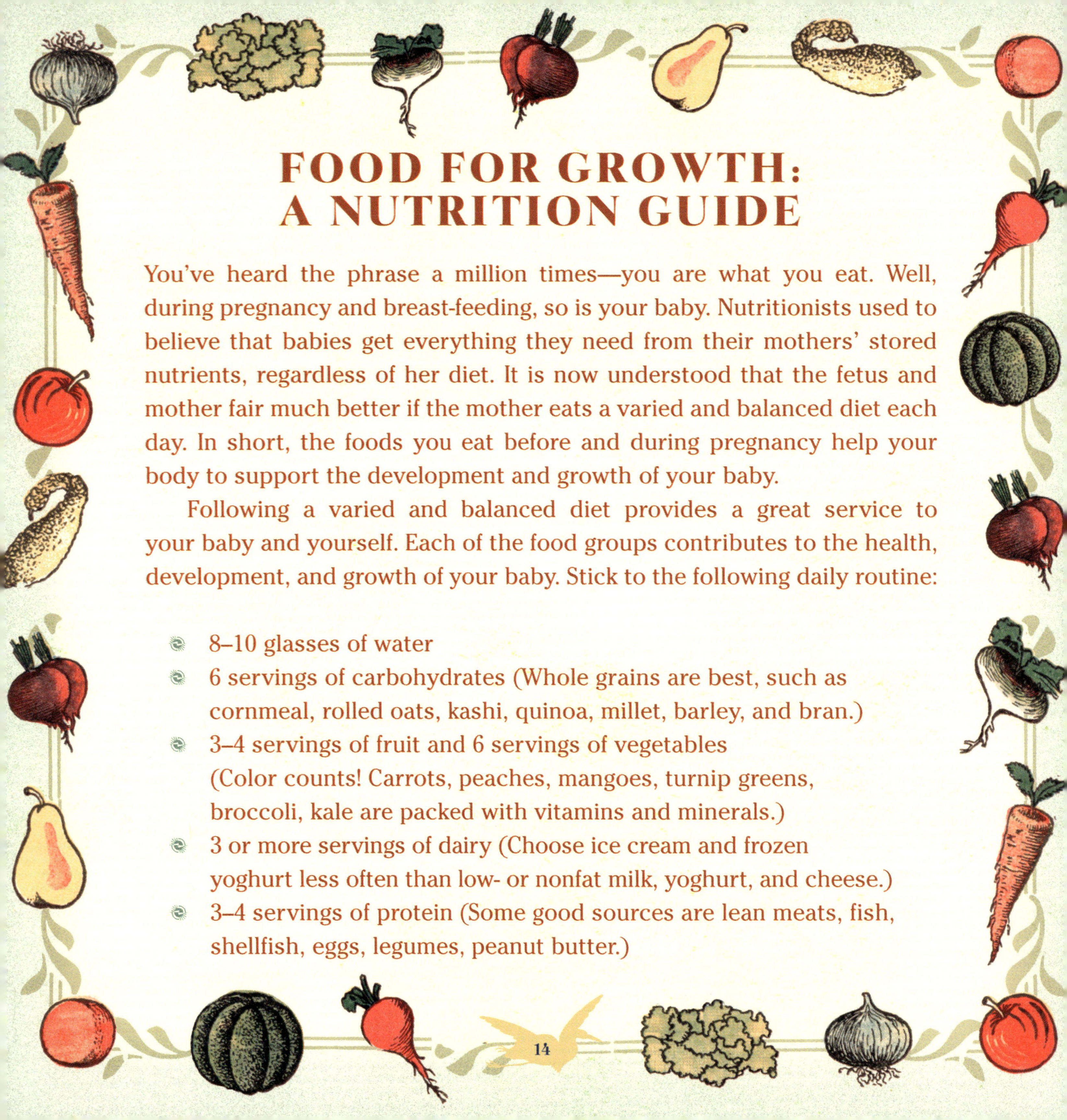

FOOD FOR GROWTH: A NUTRITION GUIDE

You've heard the phrase a million times—you are what you eat. Well, during pregnancy and breast-feeding, so is your baby. Nutritionists used to believe that babies get everything they need from their mothers' stored nutrients, regardless of her diet. It is now understood that the fetus and mother fair much better if the mother eats a varied and balanced diet each day. In short, the foods you eat before and during pregnancy help your body to support the development and growth of your baby.

Following a varied and balanced diet provides a great service to your baby and yourself. Each of the food groups contributes to the health, development, and growth of your baby. Stick to the following daily routine:

- 8–10 glasses of water
- 6 servings of carbohydrates (Whole grains are best, such as cornmeal, rolled oats, kashi, quinoa, millet, barley, and bran.)
- 3–4 servings of fruit and 6 servings of vegetables (Color counts! Carrots, peaches, mangoes, turnip greens, broccoli, kale are packed with vitamins and minerals.)
- 3 or more servings of dairy (Choose ice cream and frozen yoghurt less often than low- or nonfat milk, yoghurt, and cheese.)
- 3–4 servings of protein (Some good sources are lean meats, fish, shellfish, eggs, legumes, peanut butter.)

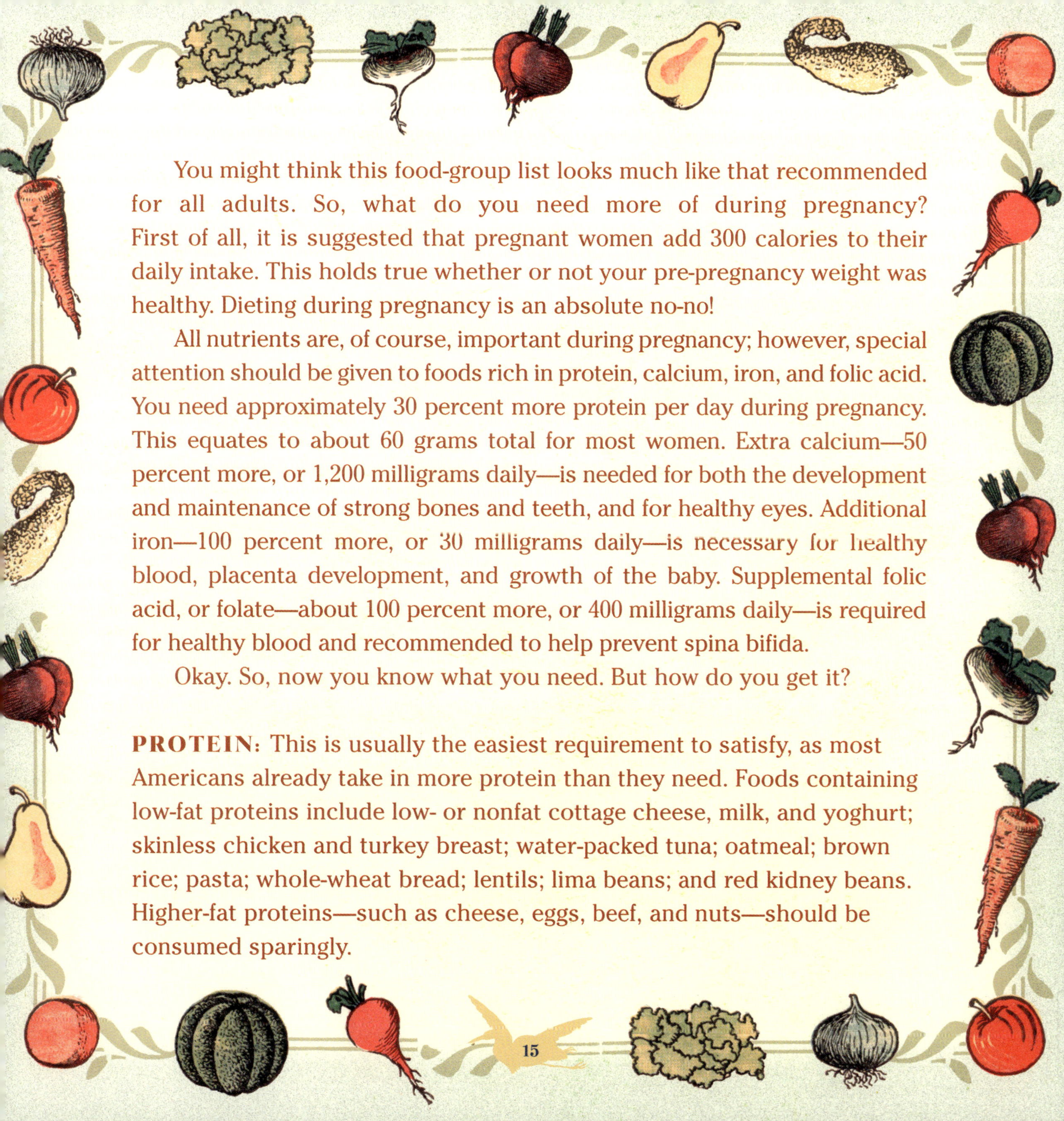

You might think this food-group list looks much like that recommended for all adults. So, what do you need more of during pregnancy? First of all, it is suggested that pregnant women add 300 calories to their daily intake. This holds true whether or not your pre-pregnancy weight was healthy. Dieting during pregnancy is an absolute no-no!

All nutrients are, of course, important during pregnancy; however, special attention should be given to foods rich in protein, calcium, iron, and folic acid. You need approximately 30 percent more protein per day during pregnancy. This equates to about 60 grams total for most women. Extra calcium—50 percent more, or 1,200 milligrams daily—is needed for both the development and maintenance of strong bones and teeth, and for healthy eyes. Additional iron—100 percent more, or 30 milligrams daily—is necessary for healthy blood, placenta development, and growth of the baby. Supplemental folic acid, or folate—about 100 percent more, or 400 milligrams daily—is required for healthy blood and recommended to help prevent spina bifida.

Okay. So, now you know what you need. But how do you get it?

PROTEIN: This is usually the easiest requirement to satisfy, as most Americans already take in more protein than they need. Foods containing low-fat proteins include low- or nonfat cottage cheese, milk, and yoghurt; skinless chicken and turkey breast; water-packed tuna; oatmeal; brown rice; pasta; whole-wheat bread; lentils; lima beans; and red kidney beans. Higher-fat proteins—such as cheese, eggs, beef, and nuts—should be consumed sparingly.

CALCIUM: The best sources of calcium are dairy products, like milk, cheese, and yoghurt. Choose low- or nonfat varieties of these foods. There are also some excellent nondairy sources of calcium: leafy green vegetables (the best are turnip greens, broccoli, and spinach), canned salmon, tofu, rhubarb, and nuts.

IRON: Foods rich in iron include lean red meats, dried beans and peas, dried fruit, and fortified cereals. Iron derived from plant foods is best absorbed if eaten in conjunction with foods rich in Vitamin C.

FOLIC ACID: A folate supplement of 0.4 milligrams per day often is recommended before and during pregnancy. There are, however, some good food sources of folate, including dark green lettuce, green peas, green beans, broccoli, dried peas and beans, oranges, and melons.

So, what shouldn't you consume during pregnancy? Some foods and substances to avoid—high-fat snacks, sugar, sodium, drugs, cigarettes, and alcohol—are obvious. But there are other foods, some of which are ordinarily considered healthy, that can cause harm to your growing baby:

- Undercooked or raw meat, poultry, eggs, or fish, which can contain bacteria
- Smoked or cured meats and fish containing sodium nitrate
- Unpasteurized dairy products or juices
- Meats and fish with a high mercury content
- Caffeine
- Sugar substitutes

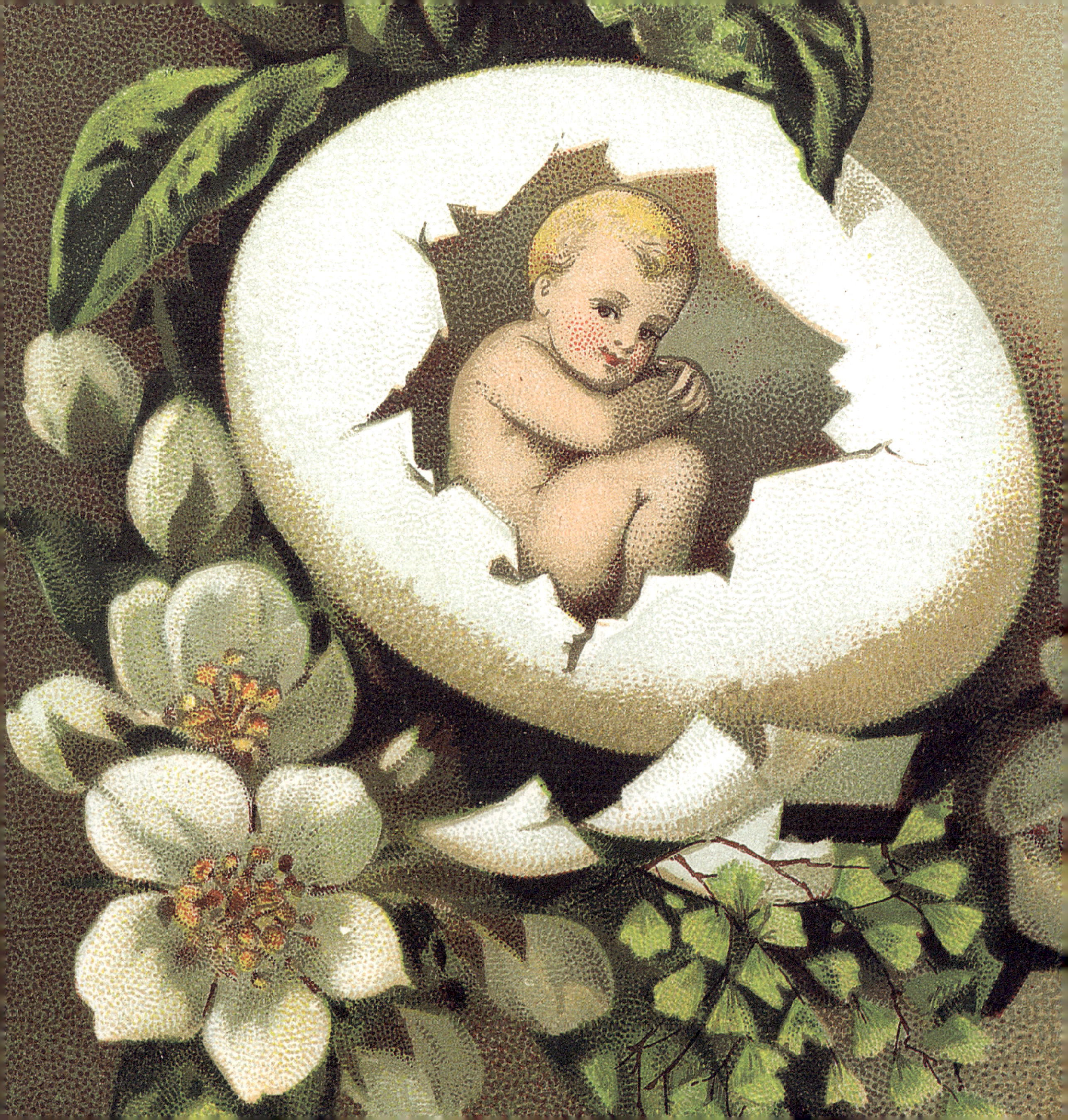

Why, when I was told the news,
I felt wings upon my shoes
And gallivanted down the street
Wanting to be indiscreet
And shout to all the world that
I
Was about to multiply.

–Dorothy Keeley Aldis

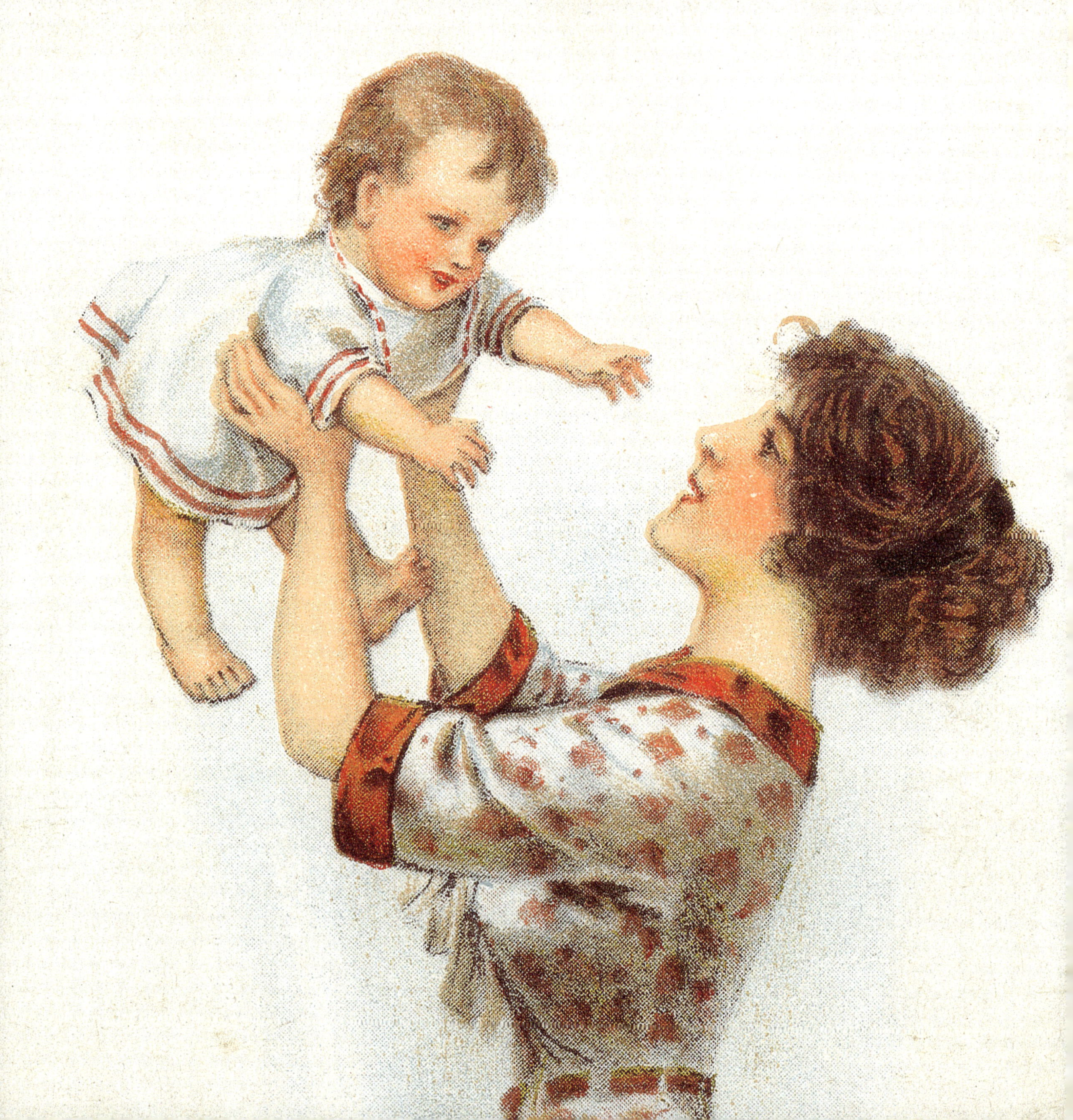

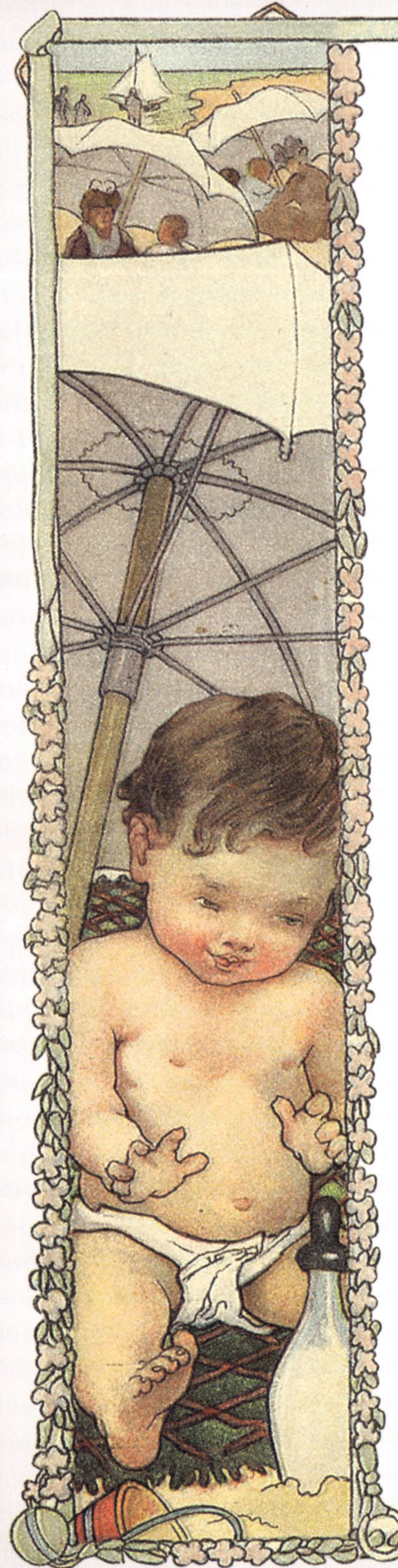

PREGNANCY FACTS

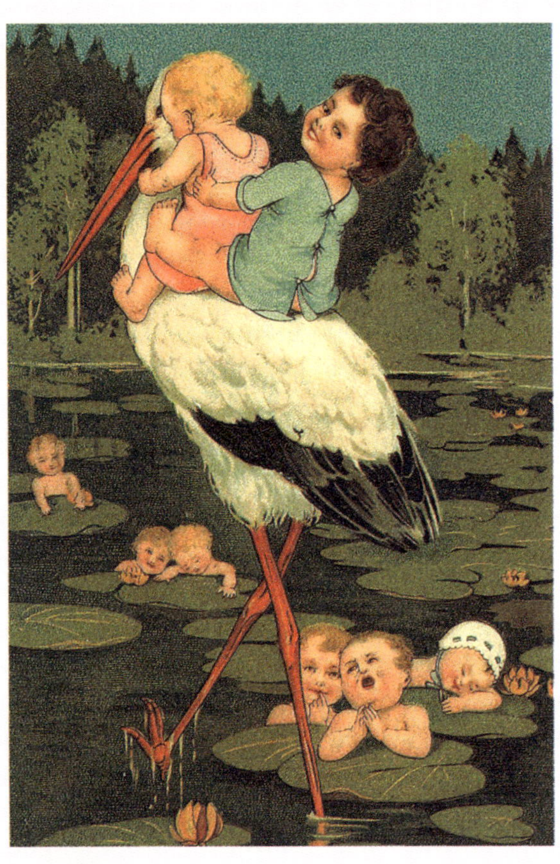

The salty fluid inside the amniotic sac protects the embryo not only from shocks, but from gravity as well. To see how this works, drop an egg still in the shell into a mayonnaise jar full of water, and shake it around.

On the 22nd day after conception the baby develops a heartbeat.

At the end of the first month of pregnancy, the baby is smaller than a grain of rice.

During pregnancy, a woman's blood volume increases nearly 50 percent.

During the course of a typical pregnancy, a woman's uterus will expand up to 20 times its normal size.

In the womb, amniotic fluid is completely recirculated by the baby every three hours.

By the ninth week, the head comprises about half of the fetus, but its growth will now slow down compared to the rest of the body.

By the 18th week in utero, a female fetus has her own fully formed uterus.

At 36 weeks, the baby is storing fat—which keeps him or her at about 32°F above the mother's body temperature.

By seven months of age, a fetus can recognize his/her mother's voice.

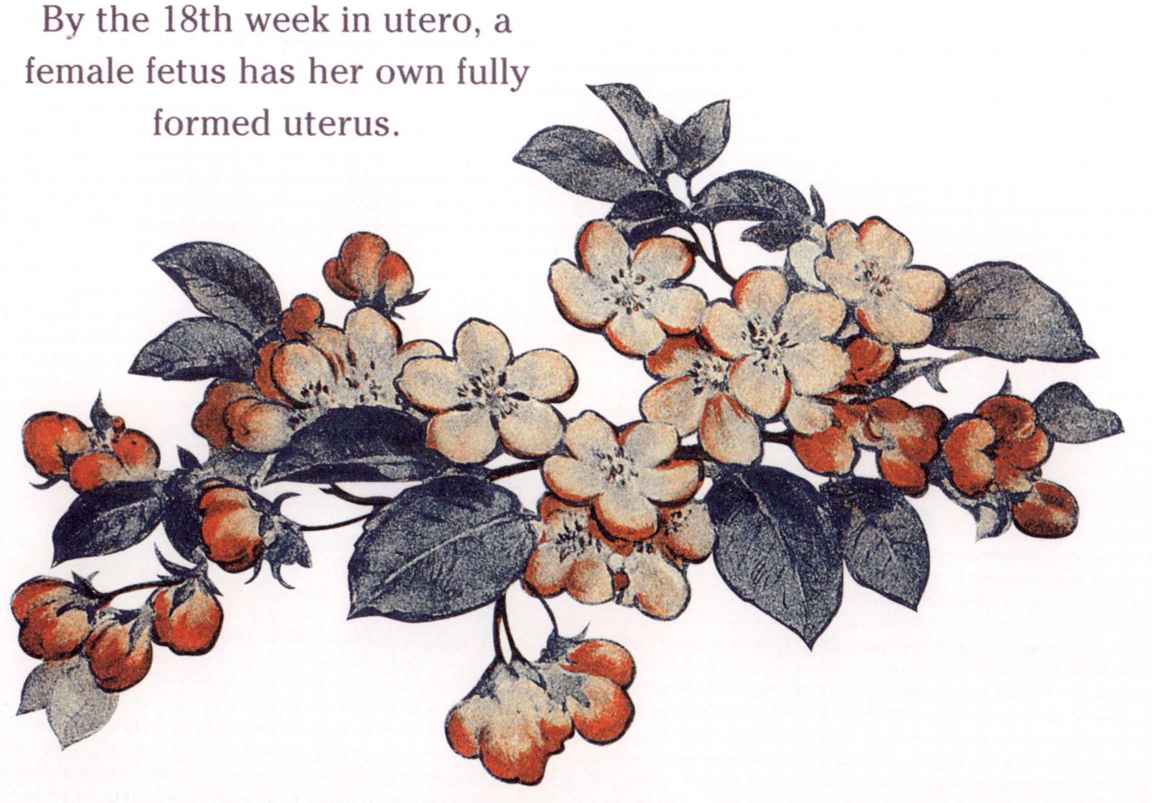

Home Remedies: *Morning Sickness*

Contrary to myth, no culture is immune to the "joys" of morning sickness. Papyrus texts show people understood unexpected nausea as far back as 2000 B.C. Women and caregivers, from the African !Kung San tribe to the Greek physician Hippocrates, have long recognized morning sickness as one of pregnancy's earliest signs.

While it often strikes at dawn, morning sickness is in no way confined to the morning. Most non-Westerners don't even use "morning" to describe the symptoms. Cantonese expectant mothers have a "pregnancy response." Russians display a "pregnancy indisposition." And in Korea, pregnant women simply enjoy "fake vomiting."

Whatever the name, 60–80 percent of all pregnant women experience strong food, drink, and smell aversions and/or vomiting, typically from week 4 through week 12. The cause is still unclear: Some believe the symptoms stem from an increase in pregnancy hormones, low blood sugar, or higher bile secretion. Others think the food and smell aversions actually serve a biological purpose, protecting the developing baby by discouraging the mom from ingesting harmful plants and toxins.

But knowing the cause won't settle your stomach; so treat yourself to some of our soothing home remedies. Experiment. See what works for you. And remember, Old Wives' tales are told by women who survived pregnancy and lived to be chatty Old Wives!

(Note: If you vomit excessively, always call your caregiver. Dehydration can be dangerous to you *and* your baby!)

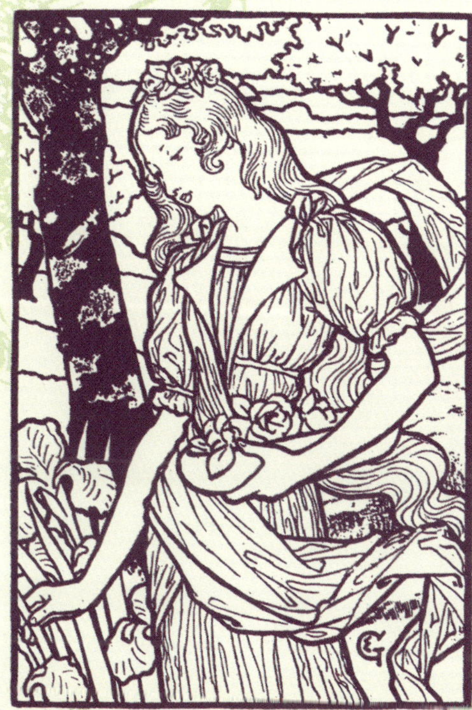

Rest & Exercise

- Try closing your eyes and lying completely still.
- Take naps, but not immediately after meals.
- Get out of bed slowly in the morning.
- Experiment with deep breathing and relaxation exercises.
- Sit and stand up straight.
- Take a walk at least once a day.
- Avoid making quick movements.

Meals & Snacks

- Eat small, frequent, high-protein, high-carbohydrate, low-fat meals. Fatty foods take longer to digest, promoting nausea.
- Eat crackers and breads made of whole grain.
- Try crunchy, salty foods.
- Avoid greasy, spicy, or smelly foods.
- If vomiting persists, try sticking with one food you know you can tolerate. Add another food each day, as your stomach allows.
- Eat whatever you can keep down whenever you want it. Better to eat less than ideally than not gain the needed weight.
- Keep a snack by your bed to eat before you get up.
- Always keep a little food in your stomach; nausea occurs more frequently on an empty stomach.
- Snack often on dry, high-carbohydrate foods (crackers, vanilla wafers, toast, cereals). They go down easily and stay down.
- Try frozen popsicles, fruit sorbets, ice cream, yoghurt, or milk shakes.

Drinks

- Drink between, instead of with, meals.
- Drink small amounts of fluids regularly to avoid dehydration—up to 12 glasses a day.
- Drink non-caffeinated teas, like peppermint, ginger root, and chamomile.
- Try room-temperature drinks or "flat" sodas.
- Try sucking on ice chips.
- Try milk sweetened with sugar or pasteurized honey.
- Dissolve wheat germ in warm milk; try sipping a few teaspoons hourly.

Herbs/Supplements

(Always consult your caregiver before trying any of these!)

- Suck on peppermint candies. Be sure candy is made with real peppermint oil and not artificial flavoring.
- Try taking your prenatal vitamins later in the day (or talk to your caregiver about temporarily stopping your prenatals to see if nausea eases; you may still need to take folic acid.)
- Talk to your caregiver about changing your iron supplement. Iron can be rough on your stomach..

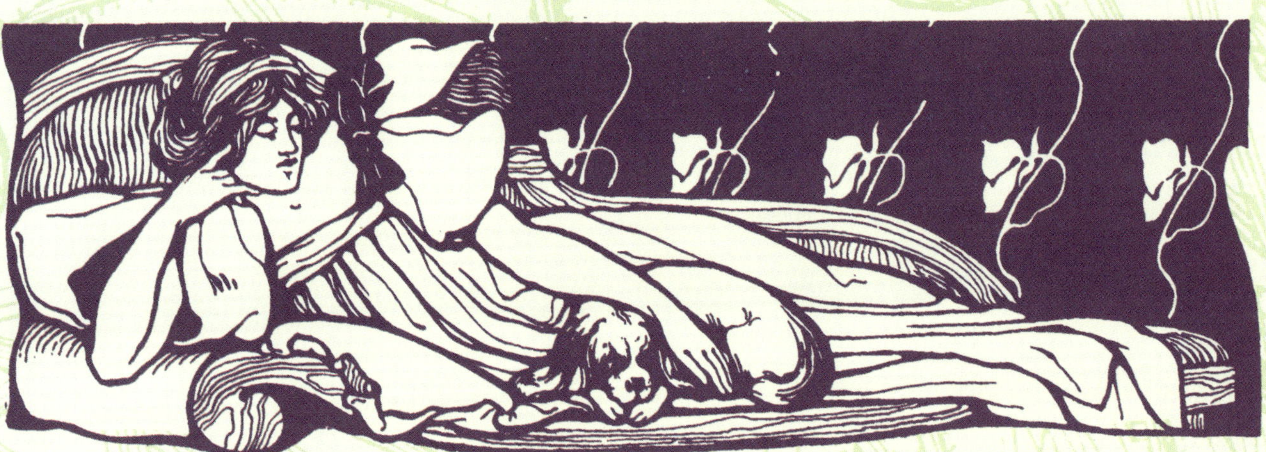

Aromatherapy

- Sniff a fresh lemon peel.
- Drip 3 drops lavender oil and 1 drop peppermint oil into a diffuser to freshen the air.
- Put a cool, lavender-scented cloth on your forehead and a warm lavender compress over your chest.
- Make sure you breathe as much fresh air as possible.

Triggers

(If reading this makes you sick, skip it!)

- Avoid strong odors, like coffee, fish, onions, garlic, garbage, vitamins, perfume, cigarette smoke, dirty diapers, gas fumes, room fresheners, and cleaning products.
- If you can't escape a noxious smell, breathe through a tissue pre-dipped in a non-nauseating essential oil such as lemon, grapefruit, ginger, or spearmint.
- Turn on fans and open windows when you cook.
- Cook with a microwave to minimize smells.
- Avoid cooking by eating prepackaged meals.
- Try eating more cold foods; they often have less nauseating odors.
- Tank up at full-service gas stations.

Some Other Good Ideas

- Don't brush your teeth right after a meal.
- Wear motion sickness wristbands to stimulate acupressure points.
- Try meditation and yoga to relax your mind and body.
- Try chewing gum.
- Stay away from warm places; higher temperatures can increase nausea.

Nothing great is created suddenly
any more than a bunch
of grapes or a fig. If you tell me
that you desire a fig, I answer you
that there must be time.
Let it first blossom, then bear fruit,
then ripen.

–Epictetus

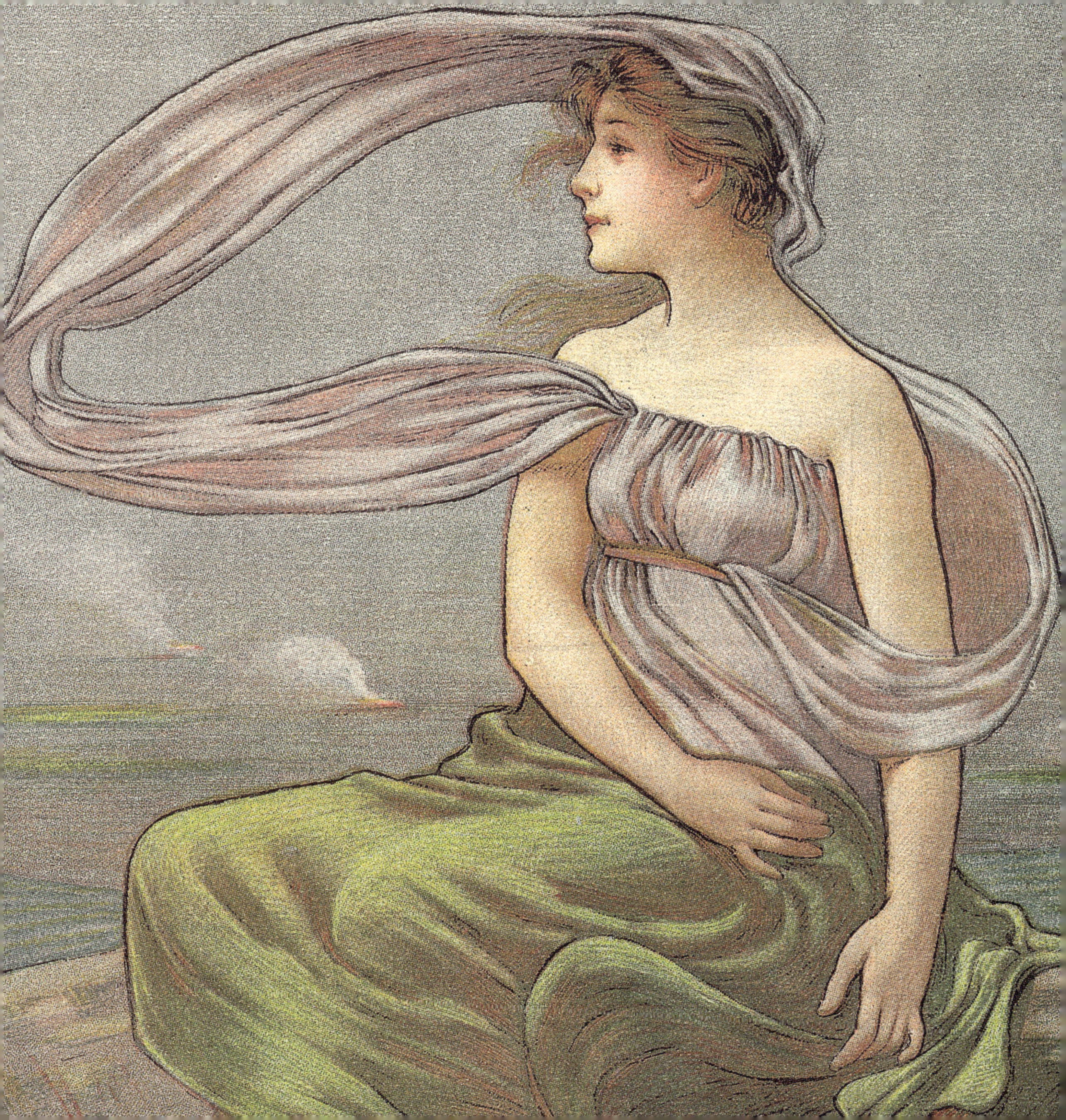

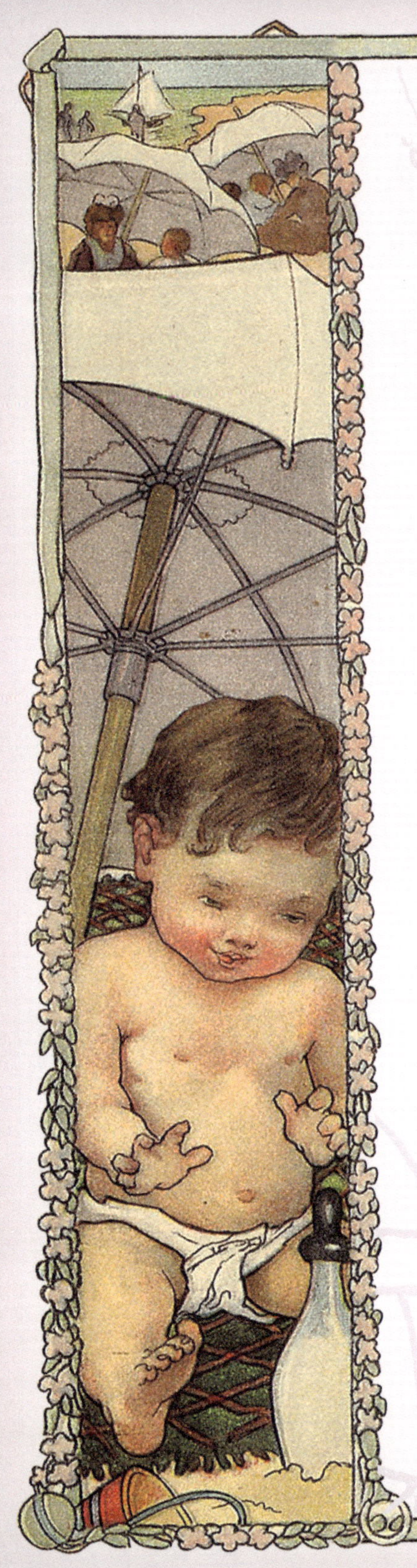

Baby Facts

Fifteen percent of a full-term baby's body is composed of fat. Eighty percent is located beneath the skin and twenty percent around the organs.

A typical newborn doubles his weight after 6 months, and triples it in a year.

A newborn baby's head accounts for about one-fourth of her entire body weight.

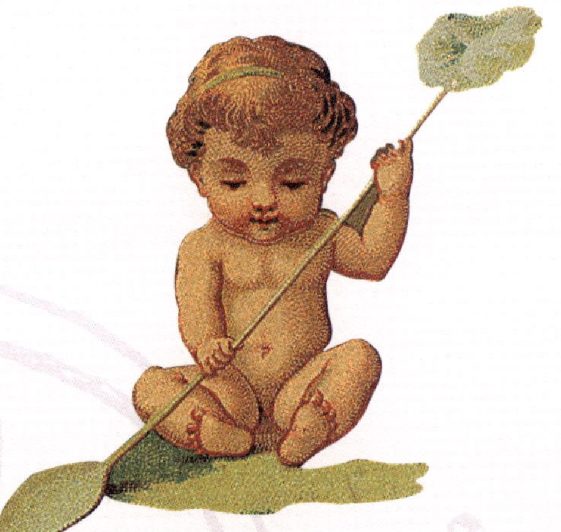

Scientists think that newborns, born with poor vision, learn to recognize their mothers by scent.

While many babies are born with blue eyes, the color may change over the next 9 months as pigment develops in the iris.

Babies can't produce tears until they are around 3–6 weeks old.

Babies are born with 300 bones, but they fuse into 206 by the time they are adults.

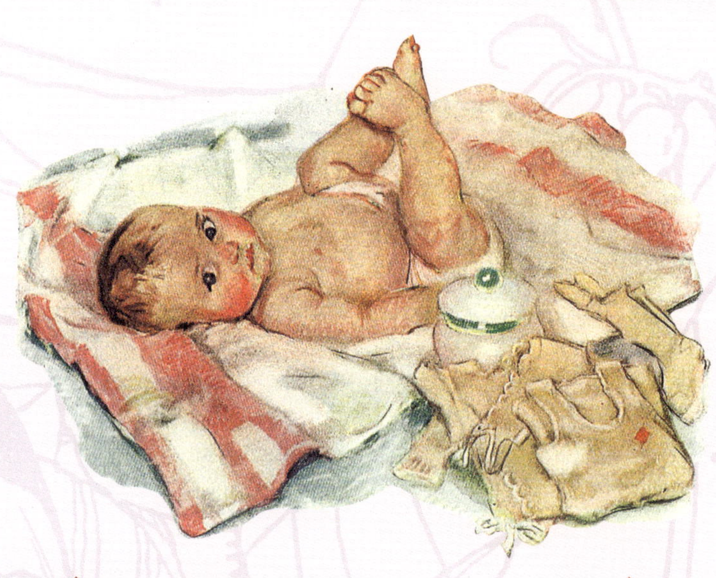

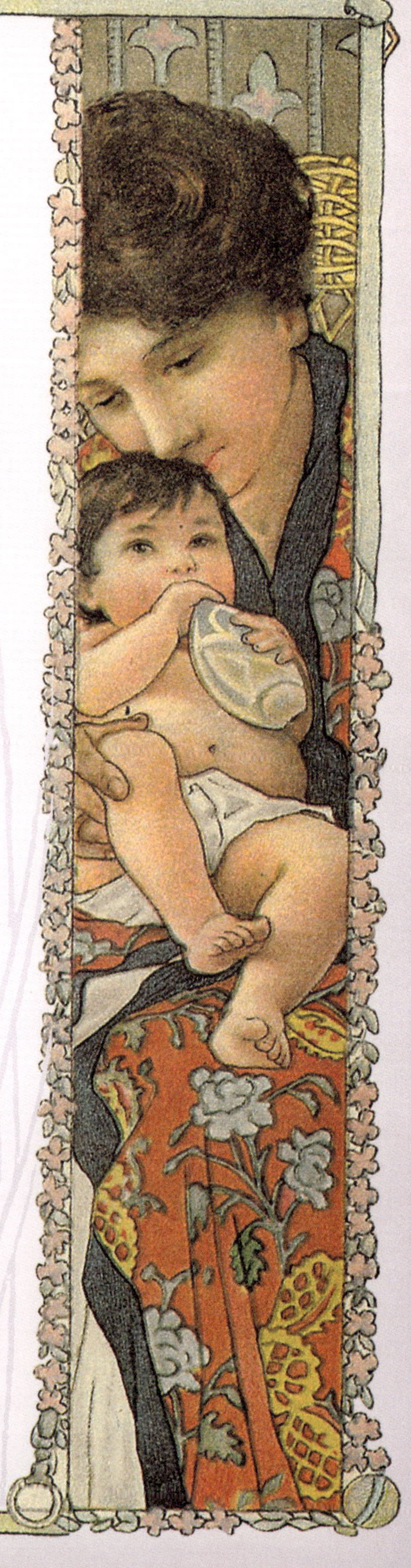

Babies born in the month of May weigh an average of 200 grams more than babies born in any other month.

Newborns have more than half a million hair follicles covering their skin.

Babies are born with fully grown fingernails and toenails, but no tear ducts.

At birth, touch is the baby's most well developed sense.

For several weeks after his birth, a baby will still assume the same fetal position it had in the womb—his muscles are used to it.

Babies are born with a "swimming reflex," and can naturally hold their breath underwater and make graceful swimming motions. They soon lose this ability, however. Some believe it may trace back to a semi-aquatic phase in recent human evolution.

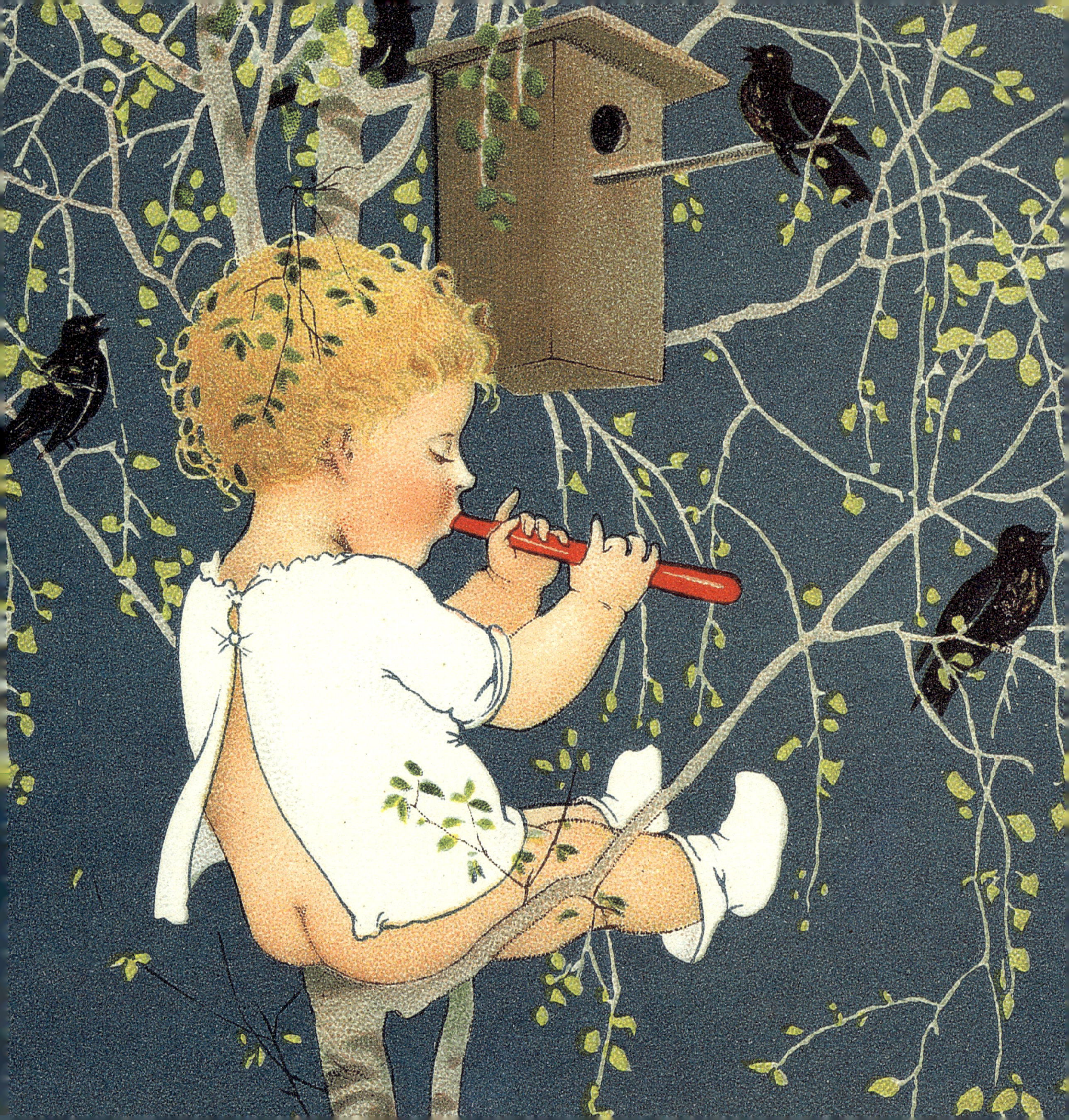

TRADITIONS: *Music & Lullabies*

Music has forever been a part of our joyous occasions and celebrations. In many cultures, it plays a pivotal role in pregnancy, birth, and child rearing. Western authorities on the subject often recommend playing classical melodies to stimulate your unborn baby and shorten labor.

In India during a Parsi ritual called *Agharni*, which takes place after the seventh month of pregnancy, relatives gather to worship, present gifts, and sing to the mother-to-be. Navaho medicine people traditionally chant and, when necessary, sing "unraveling" songs to help with labor and coax the baby out. A long-held belief by Englanders purports that the ringing of church bells helps to ease a baby's birth. A call-and-response song used in the Central African Republic during delivery goes, *Ei-oh mother of mine, my belly hurts me.* The response is *Tie up your heart*, which means "Tough it out." After a baby is born in Morocco, women and children "sing the news," proclaiming to all the new birth. And in Latvia, after the baby's naming ceremony, guests and godparents attend a feast, dancing with the baby and singing songs of good wishes.

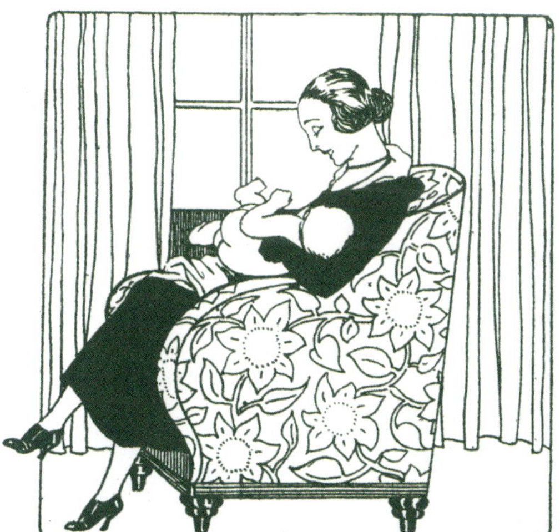

A favorite form of music the world over is the lullaby; a simple, gentle, often repetitive song that parents croon while rocking their little ones to sleep. Lullabies reassure children that everything is all right, that they are loved and cared for, and that their parents are close at hand. Some lullabies express parents' hopes and worries. Others tell stories and teach lessons. Hushed lullabies sung by the Mossi of Burkina Faso tell the baby of his or her family history, musically passing along the entire family tree.

We've gathered together some much beloved lullabies from around the world. Read through them, if only to remember the words of a favorite from childhood. Many mothers enjoy singing to their little one in the womb. And later, if you can't remember every verse, don't stop singing. Rock your baby and hum. Your loving, soothing voice is often comfort enough.

Caroline Islands, Ulithi Atoll

Float on the water,
In my arms, my arms,
On the little sea,
On the big sea,
The channel sea,
The rough sea,
The calm sea,
On this sea.

France

Are you sleeping, are you sleeping?
Brother John, Brother John?
Morning bells are ringing, morning bells
are ringing
Ding ding dong, ding ding dong.

Germany
(Johannes Brahms)

Lullaby and good night,
with roses bedight
With lilies o'er spread
is baby's wee bed
Lay thee down now and rest,
may thy slumber be blessed
Lay thee down now and rest,
may thy slumber be blessed.

Lullaby and good night,
thy mother's delight
Bright angels beside
my darling abide
They will guard thee at rest, thou
shalt wake on my breast
They will guard thee at rest, thou
shalt wake on my breast

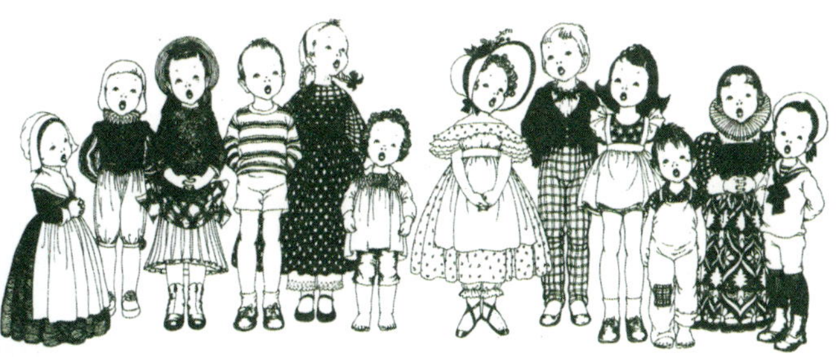

Greece
Now then sleep, sleep my child.
Sleep and dream my lovely child.
I'll give you the city of
Alexandria in sugar;
All of Cairo in rice.
And rich Constantinople.
And there you shall reign for
three years.

Haiti
Sleep mosquitoes sleep,
Sleep mosquitoes sleep.
Three hours before dawn
Mosquitoes begin to sting
I know not which position
To shift to!
Sleep mosquitoes sleep.

Hopi
Pu'va, pu'va, pu'va.
On the trail the beetles
On each others' backs are sleeping.

So on mine my baby, thou.
Pu'va, pu'va, pu'va.
Pu'va, pu'va, pu'va.

Ireland

Over in Killarney
Many years ago
Me mother sang a song to me
In tones so sweet and low.
Just a simple little ditty,
In her good old Irish way,
And I'd give the world
If she could sing
That song to me this day.

Too-ra-loo-ra-loo-ra
Too-ra-loo-ra-li
Too-ra-loo-ra-loo-ra
Hush now don't you cry
Too-ra-loo-ra-loo-ra
Too-ra-loo-ra-li
Too-ra-loo-ra-loo-ra
That's an Irish lullaby.

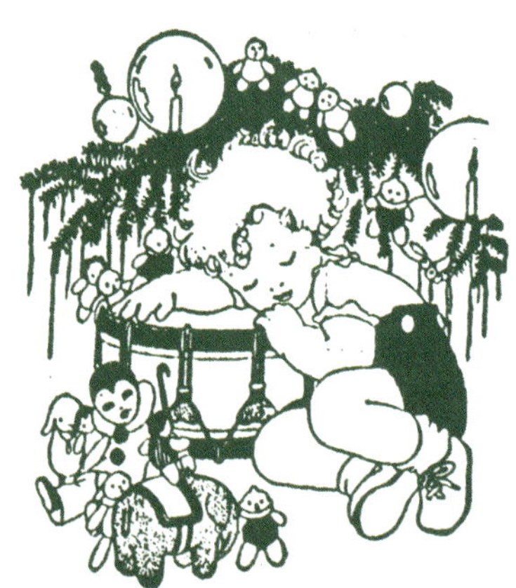

Russia

Sleep, ah sleep, my darling baby,
Su, su, lullaby.
See the moon is watching o'er thee,
Peacefully on high.
Thou shalt hear a wondrous story,
Close each wakeful eye,
And a song as well I'll sing thee,
Su, su, lullaby.

USA

Hush little baby, don't say a word.
Papa's gonna buy you a mockingbird.
And if that mockingbird won't sing,
Papa's gonna buy you a diamond
ring.
And if that diamond ring turns brass,
Papa's gonna buy you a looking
glass.
And if that looking glass gets broke,
Papa's gonna buy you a billy goat.
And if that billy goat won't pull,
Papa's gonna buy you a cart and bull.
And if that cart and bull fall down,
You'll still be the sweetest little baby
in town.

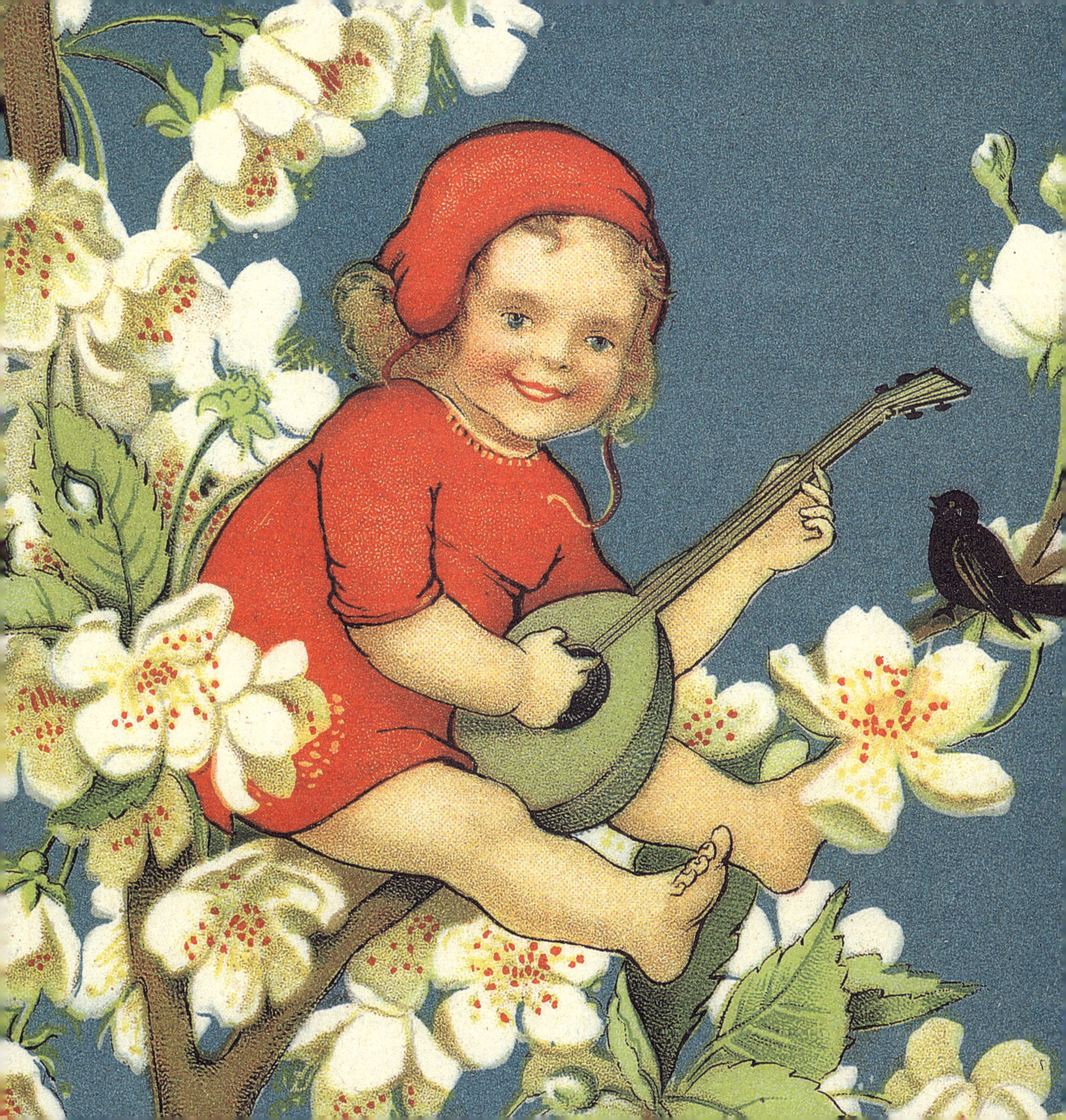

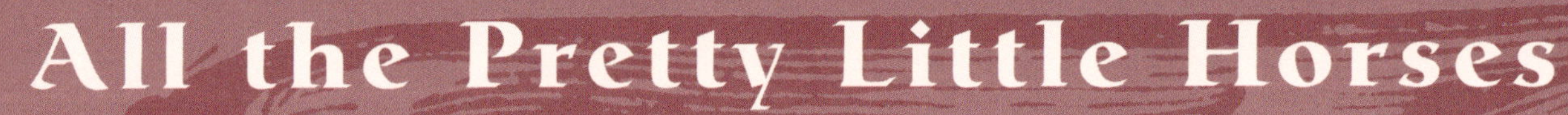

All the Pretty Little Horses

Hush-a-bye,
don't you cry.
Go to sleep-y,
little baby.
When you wake,
You shall have
all the pretty
little horses.
Blacks and bays,
dapple grays,
coach and
six white horses.

Hush-a-bye,
don't you cry,
Go to sleep-y,
little baby.

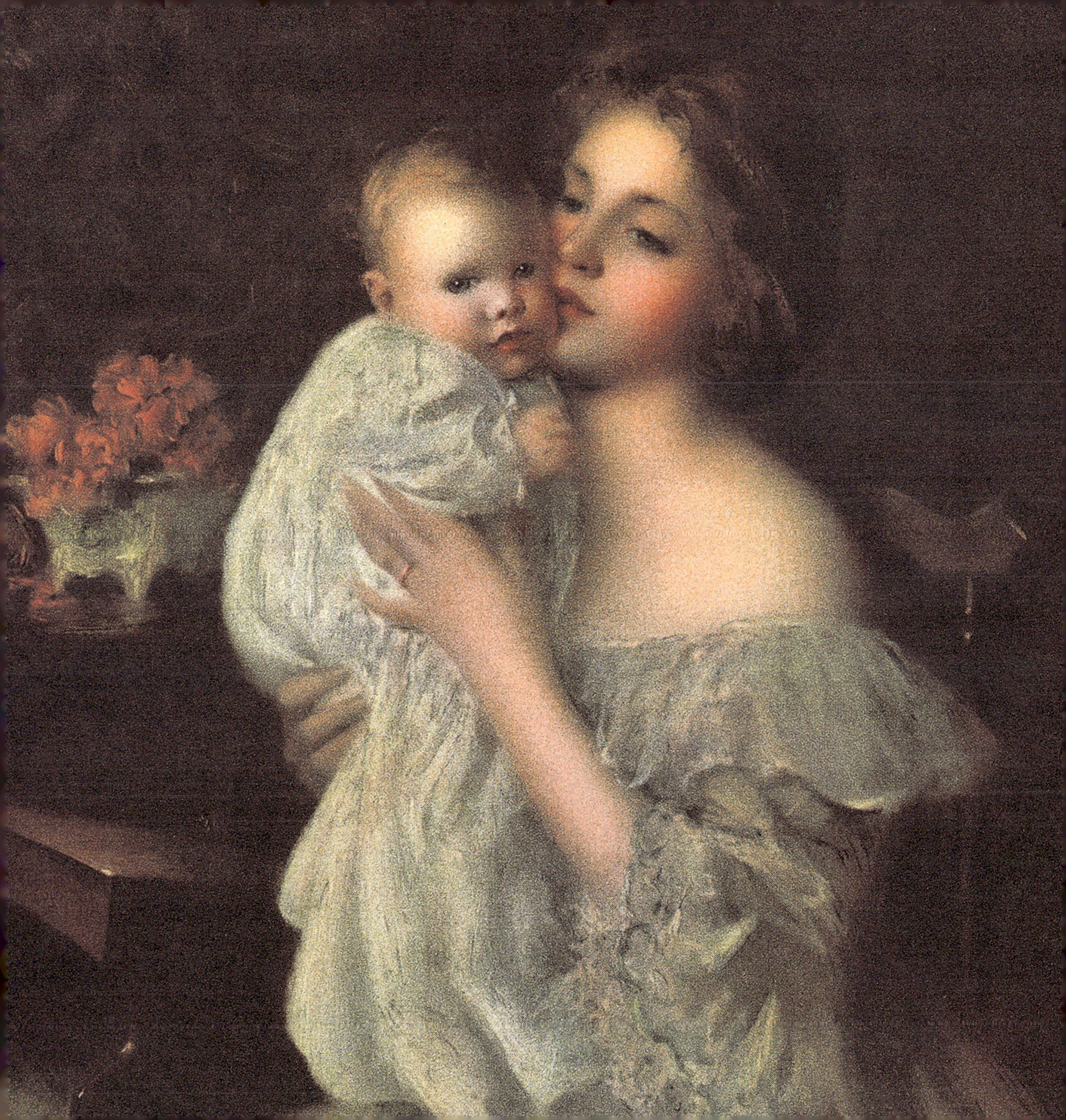

Baby Horoscopes

One of the best parts of being pregnant is imagining who that little life inside you will turn out to be. Will she be a dancer, a doctor, a musician, a teacher? Will he be witty, wild, sensitive, or serious? How about ambitious or introspective? Well, we can't give you all the answers, but we did consult the stars, and here is what they have to say....

CAPRICORN

Your child is blessed with innate wisdom beyond experience, a love of competition, and a self-deprecating sense of humor. Your bundle of joy can excel in business and politics, and develops high personal standards. Lavish this baby with lots of love and praise to help balance self-effacing tendencies. Activity that evokes laughter helps lighten that serious nature.

AQUARIUS

Your life won't be dull, since the Aquarius child is full of surprises, and has been given the courage to be an individual in a world full of conformity. Aquarians are born to overthrow the past and invent the future, so this little one loves experimenting and testing limits. Nurture that innate curiosity and the rewards will be great for both parents and child.

PISCES

Tenderhearted, intuitive, creative, with boundless imagination and the soul of a poet, your Pisces child excels in work and play activities that utilize these wonderful gifts. Water and music soothes the spirit and nurtures talent too. Trying to shield this intuitive child from unpleasant emotions or experiences is impossible, so deliver the truth, tailored to suit his age.

ARIES

Get ready for the ride of your life—this little soul is a powerhouse of energy and talents. *Active* is the keyword, and *fearless* too, so remove tall objects once climbing is mastered or attach a bungee cord for safety's sake. Innate confidence and natural leadership abilities can lead to success in a myriad of fields. Discipline is needed, but not so firm that it breaks her spirit.

TAURUS

Your little Taurus is creative, naturally easygoing, and has great common sense. She loves soft fabrics and the touch of your hand. A baby massage soothes and satisfies a little Taurus's need for physical sensation; regular routines provide security; and a love of food and drink gives him a healthy appetite. Endurance and patience are assets that can turn to stubbornness in a test of wills.

GEMINI

Curiosity personified is your precious Gemini, along with a quick wit, imagination, and intellect. A fun-loving nature makes settling down to do one thing impossible, but her ability to juggle several activities at once is innate, so handling a variety of tasks later on will be second nature. *Changeable*, *adaptable*, and *versatile* are keywords to your child's talents and happiness.

CANCER

Cancer is *the* zodiac sign for childhood, family, and home, so feelings and nurturing instincts are strong here. You can never love a Cancer child too much or too often: Like a flower, he blooms or wilts, stands tall, or clings to the vine, depending on the love he receives. Mom and Dad are everything to this little soul, and the language of the heart is the one that Cancer knows best.

LEO

Mom and Dad have every right to be proud of their little Leo, who is blessed with a sunny disposition, loving heart, abundant creativity, and instinctual leadership abilities. A natural flair for drama is an asset that can serve her well in both business and the arts—perhaps even on stage or screen. Pride is strong too, along with Leo's innate dignity, so discipline in private and praise in public.

VIRGO

Keep your running shoes handy, because this child will be in constant motion, both physically *and* mentally. An active, curious mind coupled with unlimited nervous energy keeps parents on their toes. High personal standards, including a love of order and perfection, makes Virgo a little shy or self-deprecating, so your role is to reassure him with lots of love.

LIBRA

Born with natural grace and charm, this child has a winning way *and* appearance, being usually well proportioned and attractive, with an innate sense of style that can translate to success in the arts, especially fashion, design, and architecture. On the other hand, your peace-loving and fair-minded Libra could excel in law or public relations. Encourage decisiveness early and consistently.

SCORPIO

The intense little Scorpio will do nothing halfway. Intuitive and loyal, your child will bond deeply with loved ones, and can be possessive of people and property. Sharing is hard to learn but necessary and easier if a couple of toys are set aside solely for her use. Rejection is Scorpio's greatest fear, and love is the only antidote.

SAGITTARIUS

Optimistic, idealistic, and independent, your child is always looking for the next great adventure. Fun-loving and naturally athletic, he finds more activities and interests than there is time to do them. With age you'll see an above-average intellect and a dislike of routine or discipline. The Sagittarian child is blessed with a happy-go-lucky nature that will attract good will throughout her life.

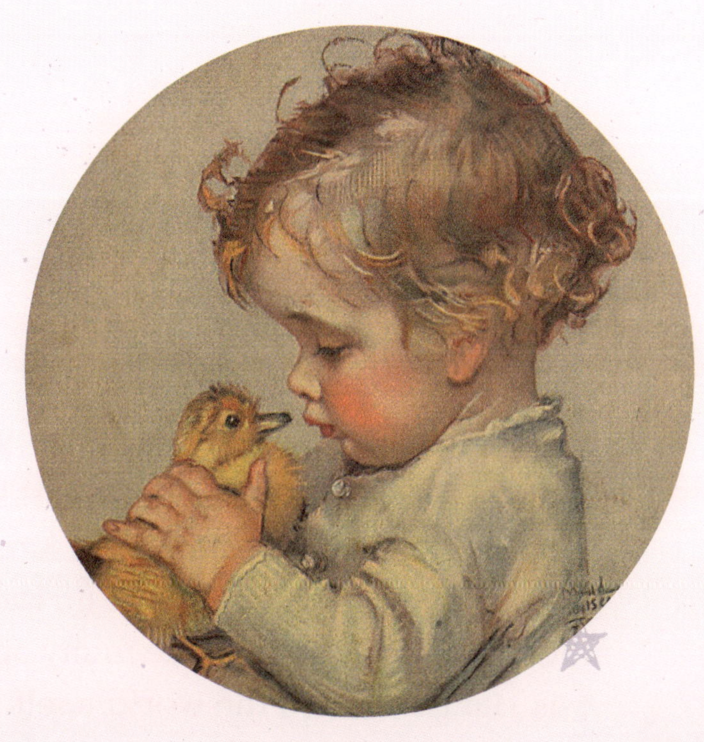

Letter to My Unborn Child

Jessie Bernard

4 May 1941

MY DEAREST,

Eleven weeks from today you will be ready for this outside world. And what a world it is this year! It has been the most beautiful spring I have ever seen. Miss Morris (a faculty colleague) says it is because I have you to look forward to. She says she has noticed a creative look on my face in my appreciation of this spring. And she is right. But also the world itself has been so particularly sweet, aglow with color. The forsythia were yellower and fuller than any I have ever seen. The lilacs were fragrant and feathery. And now the spirea, heavy with their little round blooms, stand like wonderful igloos, a mass of white. I doff my scientific mantle long enough to pretend that Nature is outdoing herself to prepare this earth for you. But also I want to let all this beauty get into my body.

I have so many dreams for you. There are so many virtues I would endow you with if I could. First of all, I would make you tough and strong. And how I have labored at that! I have eaten vitamins and minerals instead of food. Gallons of milk, pounds of

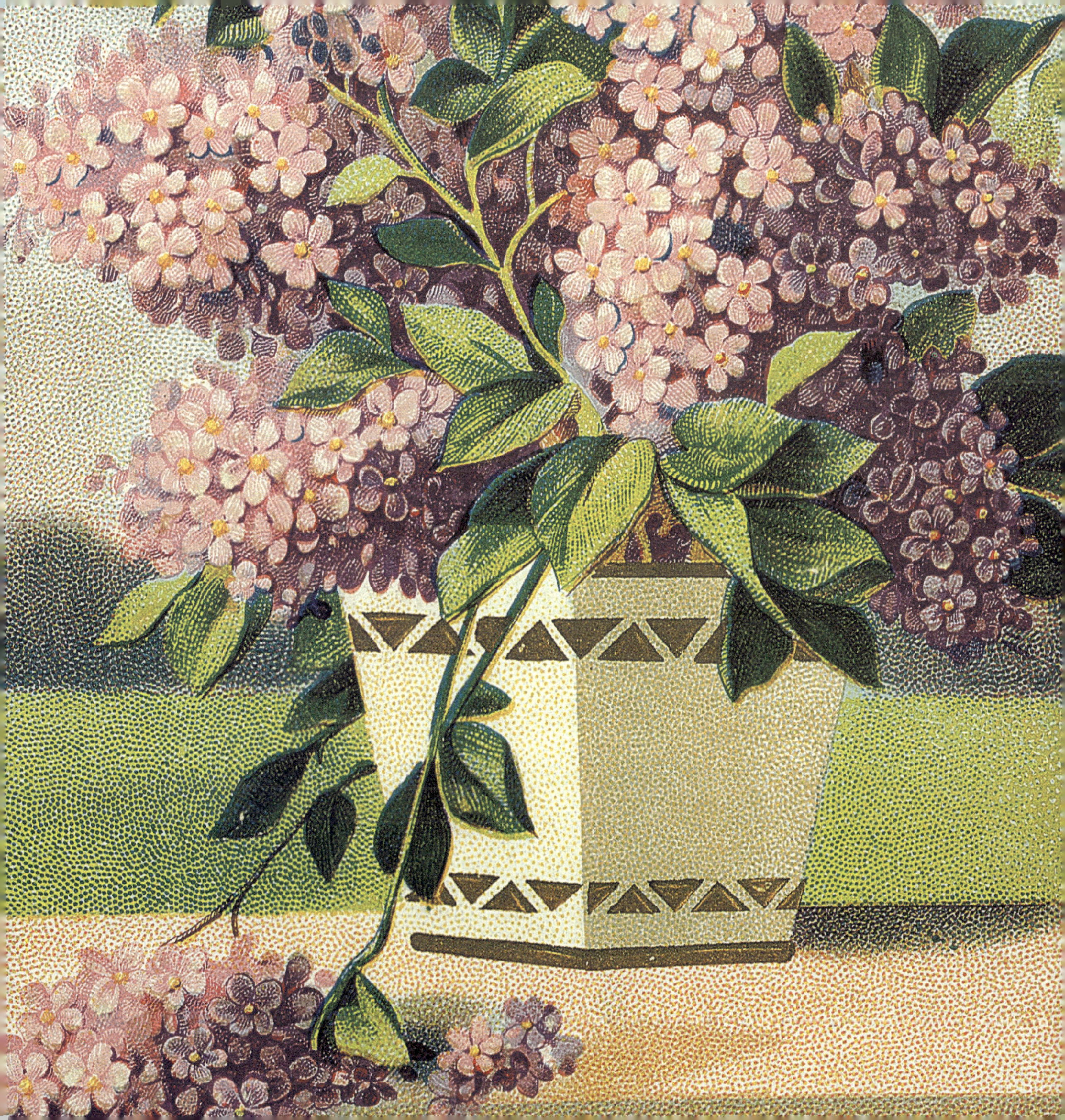

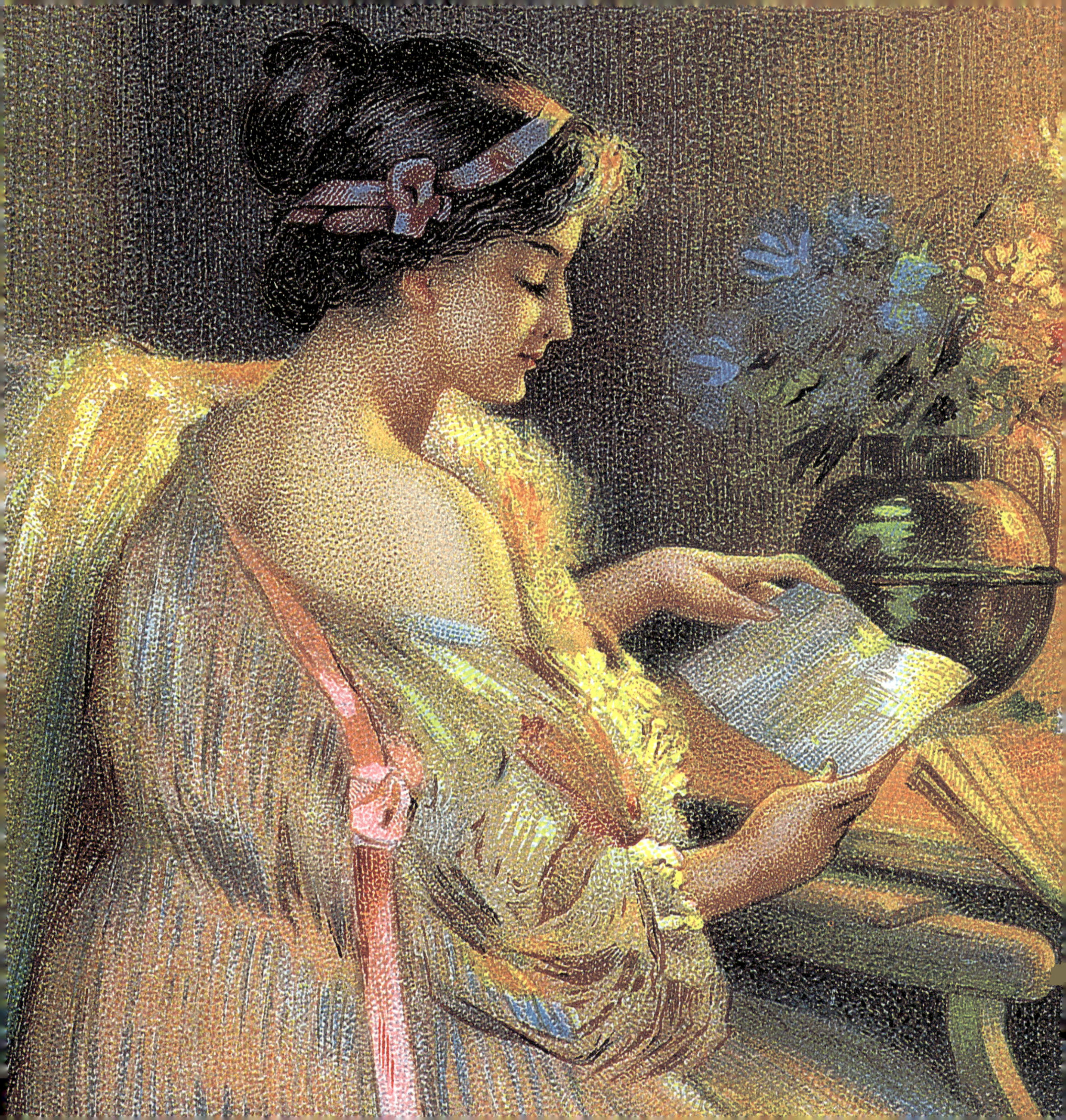

Letter to My Unborn Child

lettuce, dozens of eggs...Hours of sunshine. To make your body a strong one because everything [depends] on that. I would give you resiliency of body so that all the blows and buffets of this world would leave you still unbeaten. I would have you creative. I would have you a creative scientist. But if the shuffling genes have made of you an artist, that will make me happy too. And even if you have no special talent either artistic or scientific, I would still have you creative no matter what you do. To build things, to make things, to create—that is what I covet for you. If you have a strong body and a creative mind you will be happy. I will help in that. Already I can see how parents long to shield their children from disappointments and defeat. But I also know that I cannot re-make life for you. You will suffer. you will have moments of disappointment and defeat. You will have your share of buffeting. I cannot spare you that. But I hope to help you be such a strong, radiant, self-integrated person that you will take all this in your stride, assimilate it, and rise to conquer...

Eleven more weeks. It seems a long time. Until another time, then, my precious one, I say good-bye.

Your eager mother

Letters to Your Unborn Child

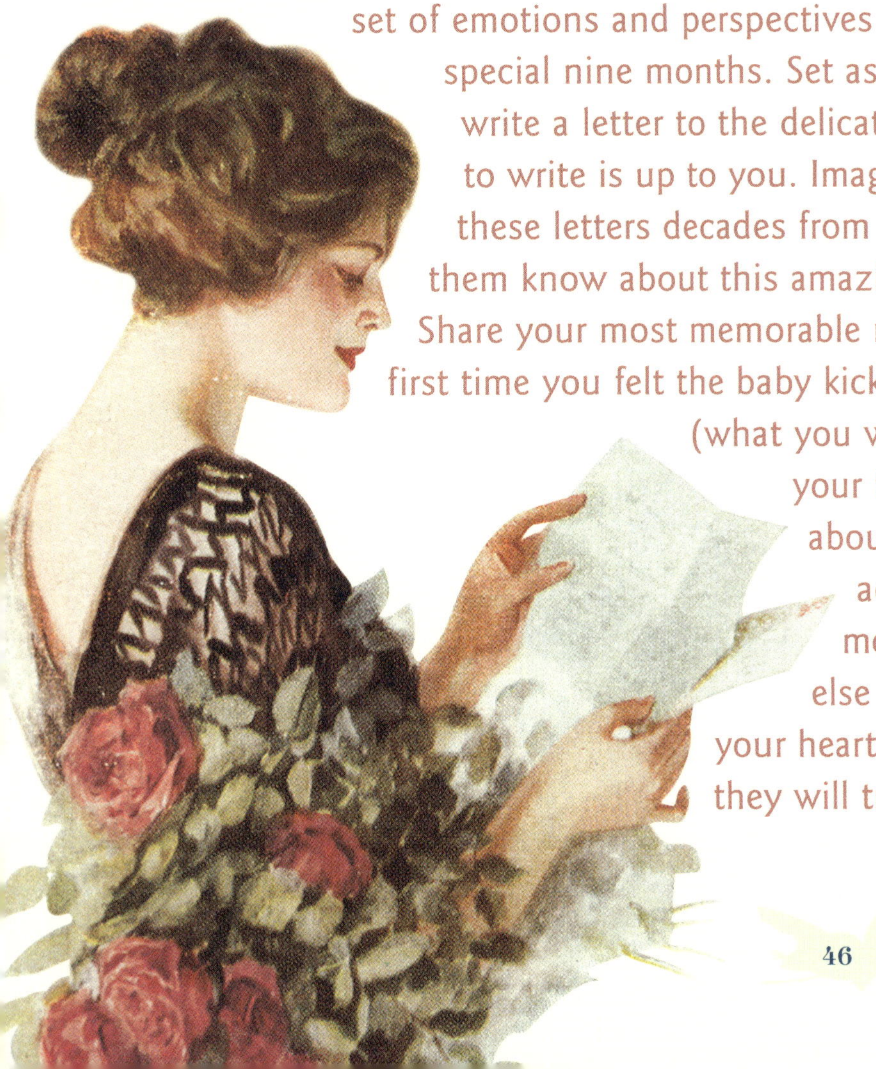

Writing to your unborn child throughout your pregnancy is a wonderful way to nurture the developing bond between you and your baby. The experience of pregnancy brings with it a whole new set of emotions and perspectives that are unique to those very special nine months. Set aside a few hours each month to write a letter to the delicate life growing inside you. What to write is up to you. Imagine your son or daughter reading these letters decades from now and imagine what you'd like them know about this amazing period in your life together. Share your most memorable moments (what it felt like the first time you felt the baby kick), your hopes for the future (what you wish for your child's happiness), your fears (what scares you most about parenthood), your wisdom and advice (what you feel are life's most important lessons), or anything else that comes to mind. Write from your heart and give your child a gift that they will treasure for a lifetime.

What To Do

- Select a beautiful set of stationery.
- Set aside ten envelopes and label nine of them "Month 1" through "Month 9." Label the tenth envelope "Your Birth."
- Encourage your partner to include a letter each month as well. While they may not be experiencing the physical aspects of pregnancy, they too are preparing to become a parent.
- Once you have finished each letter, date it and seal it in the corresponding envelope. After your baby is born, write a final letter and include the birth story. Seal it in the last envelope, labeled "Your Birth."

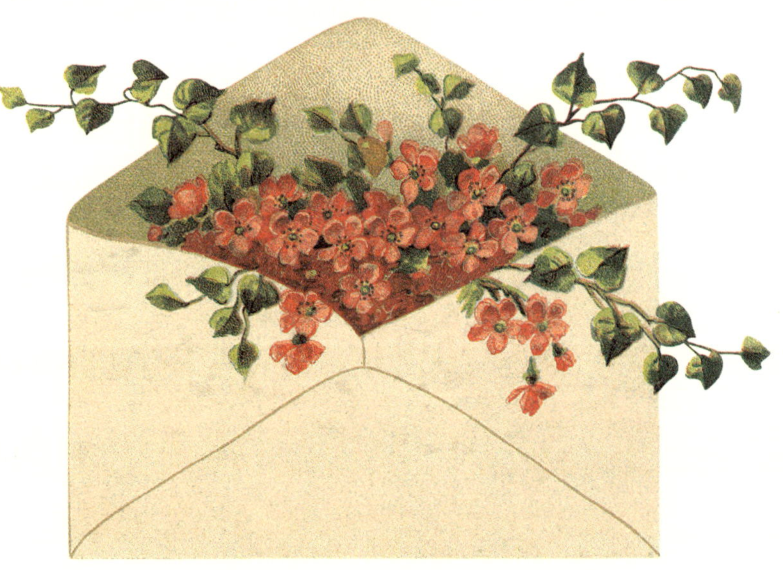

- Place the envelopes in a plastic bag and store them in a sealed acid-free box. Address the box to your child and label it "Your First Nine Months."
- Store the box in a safe and dry place until the time arrives to give this special keepsake to your son or daughter. The occasion could be a momentous birthday, like sixteen or twenty-one, or a quiet, unplanned moment that simply presents itself. Regardless of the chosen time, it will certainly be received with surprise, gratitude, joy, and love.

Often I am filled with hope; sometimes I am consumed with dread. Often I feel blessed; sometimes I feel resentful. Sometimes I am downright giddy. Sometimes I am so sentimental an AT&T commercial sends me over the edge. Sometimes I feel gorgeous, earthy, and powerful. Sometimes I feel like a helium balloon with gravity shoes...
A delusion, you say? Certainly not. Look, I'm not crazy–I'm pregnant.

–Arlene Modica Matthews

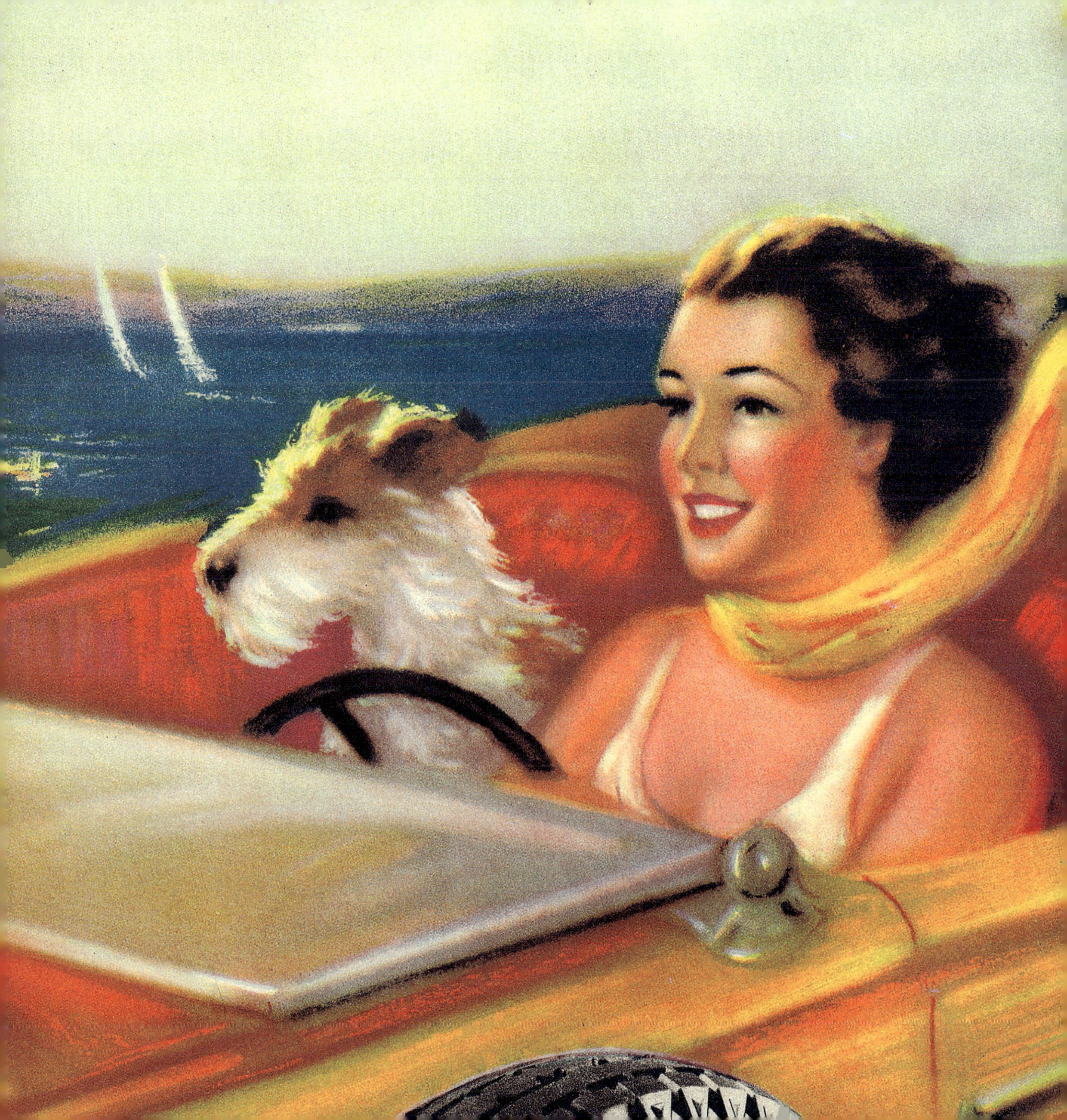

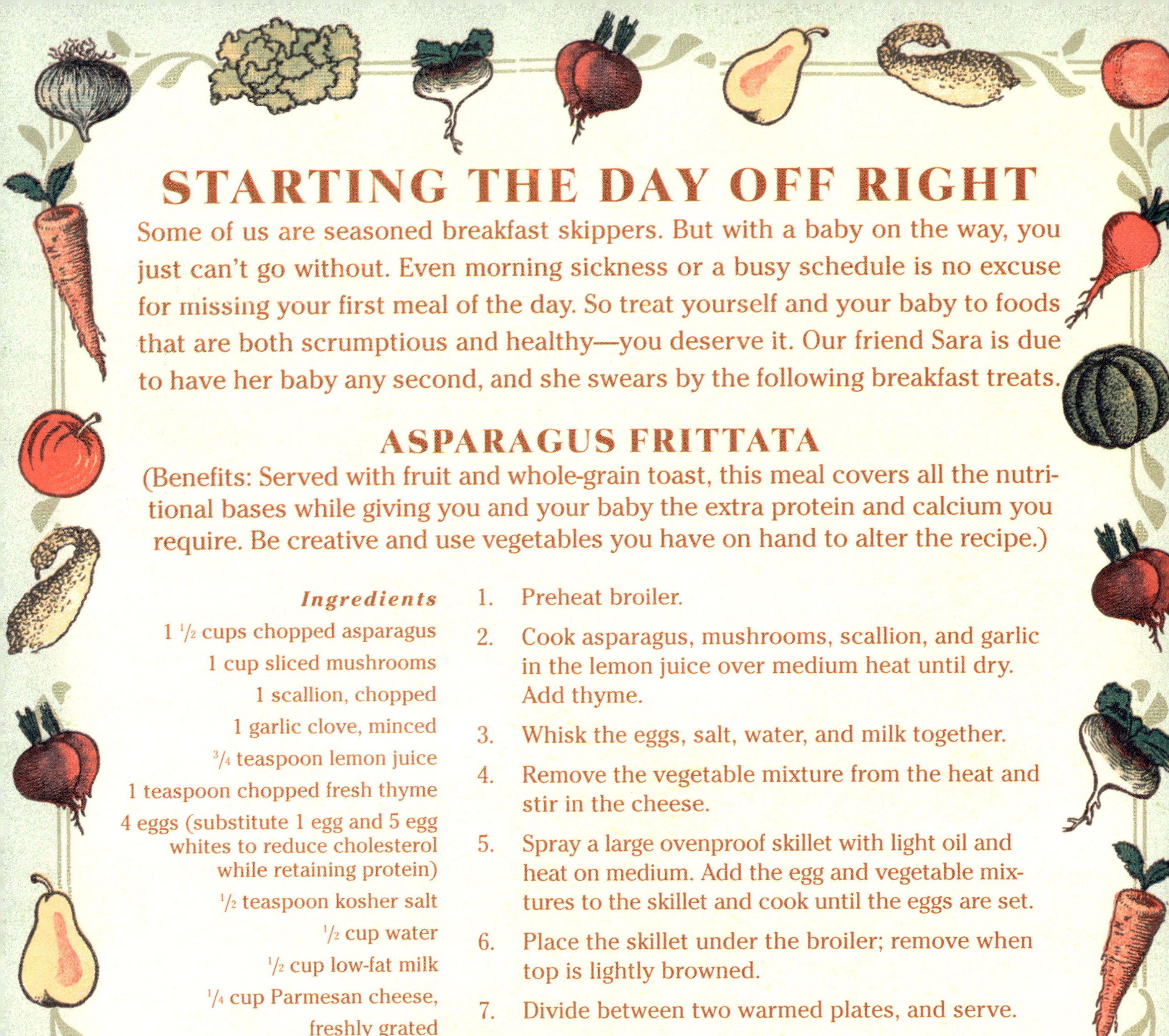

STARTING THE DAY OFF RIGHT

Some of us are seasoned breakfast skippers. But with a baby on the way, you just can't go without. Even morning sickness or a busy schedule is no excuse for missing your first meal of the day. So treat yourself and your baby to foods that are both scrumptious and healthy—you deserve it. Our friend Sara is due to have her baby any second, and she swears by the following breakfast treats.

ASPARAGUS FRITTATA

(Benefits: Served with fruit and whole-grain toast, this meal covers all the nutritional bases while giving you and your baby the extra protein and calcium you require. Be creative and use vegetables you have on hand to alter the recipe.)

Ingredients

1 ½ cups chopped asparagus
1 cup sliced mushrooms
1 scallion, chopped
1 garlic clove, minced
¾ teaspoon lemon juice
1 teaspoon chopped fresh thyme
4 eggs (substitute 1 egg and 5 egg whites to reduce cholesterol while retaining protein)
½ teaspoon kosher salt
½ cup water
½ cup low-fat milk
¼ cup Parmesan cheese, freshly grated

1. Preheat broiler.
2. Cook asparagus, mushrooms, scallion, and garlic in the lemon juice over medium heat until dry. Add thyme.
3. Whisk the eggs, salt, water, and milk together.
4. Remove the vegetable mixture from the heat and stir in the cheese.
5. Spray a large ovenproof skillet with light oil and heat on medium. Add the egg and vegetable mixtures to the skillet and cook until the eggs are set.
6. Place the skillet under the broiler; remove when top is lightly browned.
7. Divide between two warmed plates, and serve.

Serves 2.

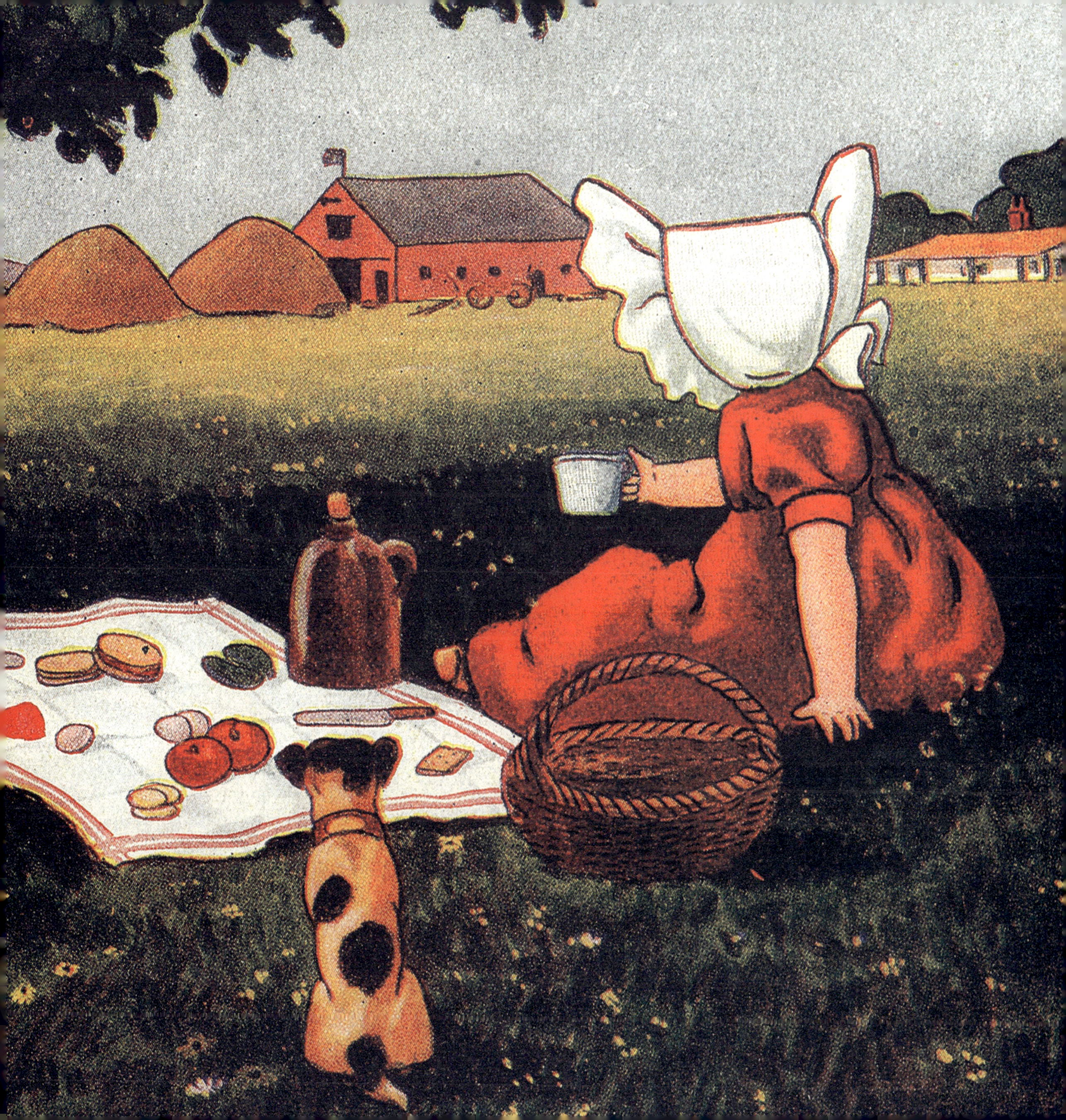

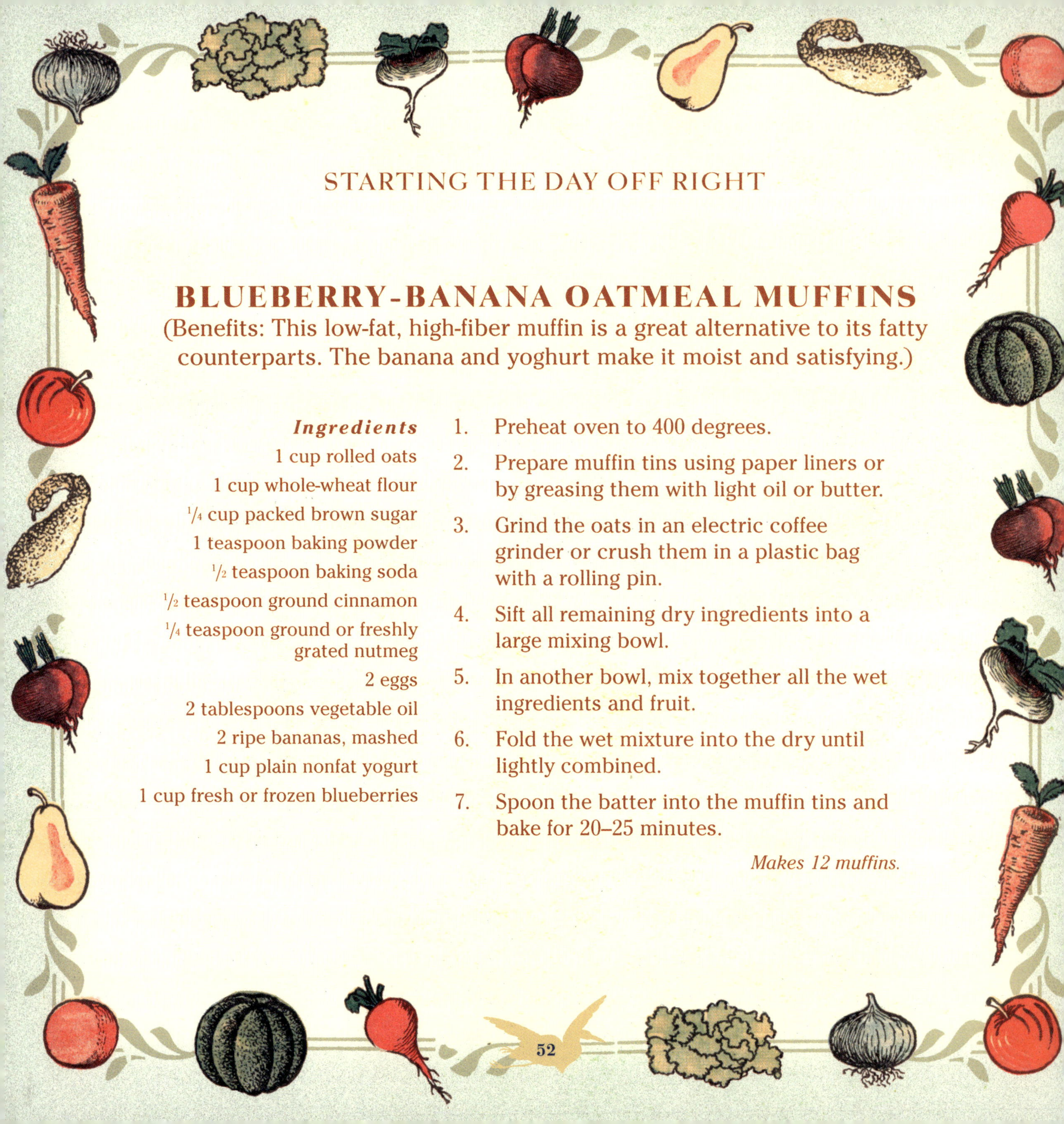

BLUEBERRY-BANANA OATMEAL MUFFINS

(Benefits: This low-fat, high-fiber muffin is a great alternative to its fatty counterparts. The banana and yoghurt make it moist and satisfying.)

Ingredients

1 cup rolled oats
1 cup whole-wheat flour
¼ cup packed brown sugar
1 teaspoon baking powder
½ teaspoon baking soda
½ teaspoon ground cinnamon
¼ teaspoon ground or freshly grated nutmeg
2 eggs
2 tablespoons vegetable oil
2 ripe bananas, mashed
1 cup plain nonfat yogurt
1 cup fresh or frozen blueberries

1. Preheat oven to 400 degrees.
2. Prepare muffin tins using paper liners or by greasing them with light oil or butter.
3. Grind the oats in an electric coffee grinder or crush them in a plastic bag with a rolling pin.
4. Sift all remaining dry ingredients into a large mixing bowl.
5. In another bowl, mix together all the wet ingredients and fruit.
6. Fold the wet mixture into the dry until lightly combined.
7. Spoon the batter into the muffin tins and bake for 20–25 minutes.

Makes 12 muffins.

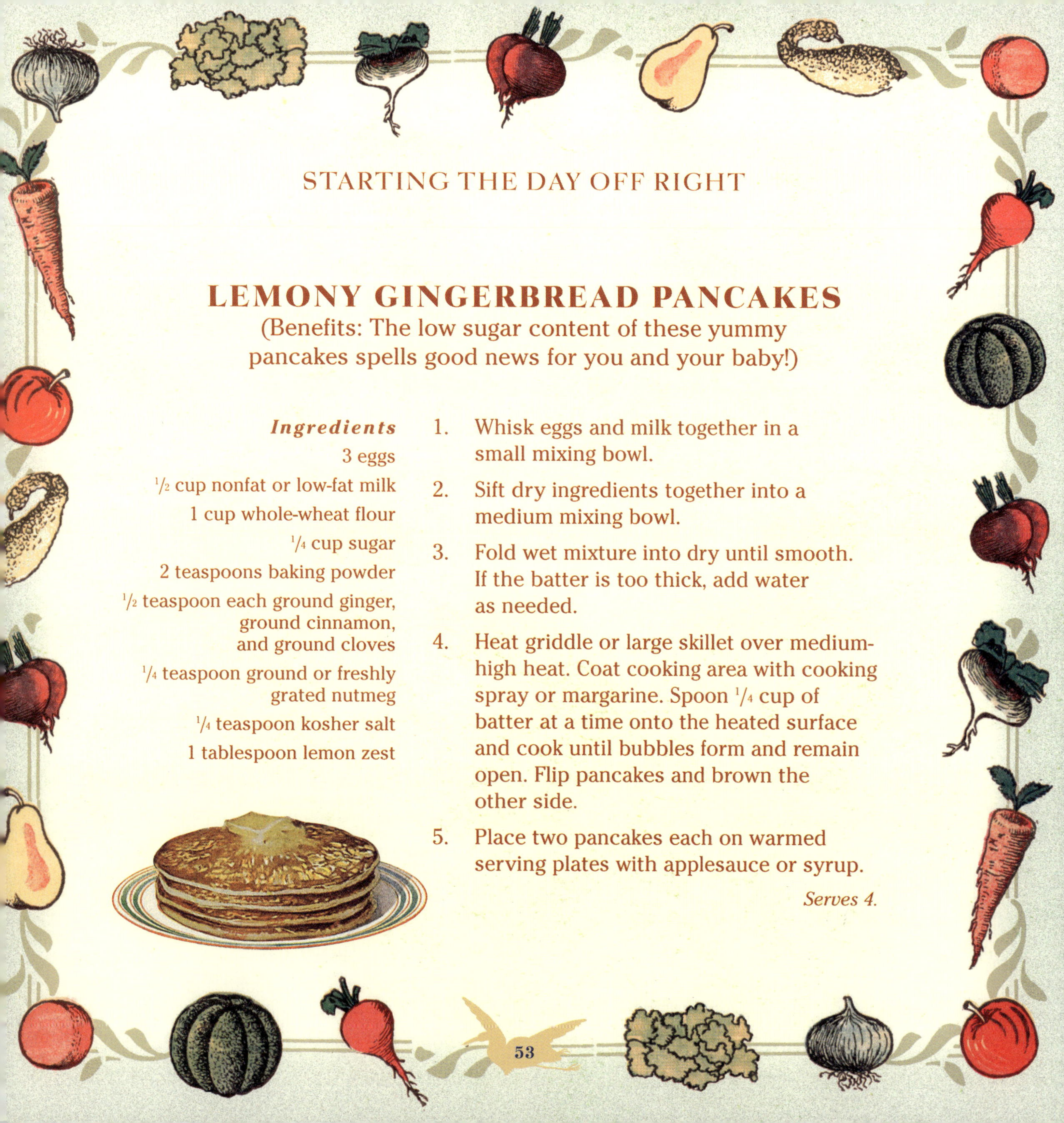

LEMONY GINGERBREAD PANCAKES

(Benefits: The low sugar content of these yummy pancakes spells good news for you and your baby!)

Ingredients

3 eggs

½ cup nonfat or low-fat milk

1 cup whole-wheat flour

¼ cup sugar

2 teaspoons baking powder

½ teaspoon each ground ginger, ground cinnamon, and ground cloves

¼ teaspoon ground or freshly grated nutmeg

¼ teaspoon kosher salt

1 tablespoon lemon zest

1. Whisk eggs and milk together in a small mixing bowl.
2. Sift dry ingredients together into a medium mixing bowl.
3. Fold wet mixture into dry until smooth. If the batter is too thick, add water as needed.
4. Heat griddle or large skillet over medium-high heat. Coat cooking area with cooking spray or margarine. Spoon ¼ cup of batter at a time onto the heated surface and cook until bubbles form and remain open. Flip pancakes and brown the other side.
5. Place two pancakes each on warmed serving plates with applesauce or syrup.

Serves 4.

Bad heartburn? Well, the good news is your baby will be born with a full head of gorgeous hair! Or at least that's what the Old Wives say. While more reliable sources may disagree with the Wives' hairy predictions, all concur that, second only to morning sickness, heartburn is a leading pregnancy complaint.

Heartburn is a burning sensation occurring in the throat and chest area, from the bottom of the breastbone to the lower throat. Pregnant women may experience heartburn at any time of the day, though it often comes on within 30 minutes of eating or at night. Symptoms may be triggered by specific foods or by overeating, exercise, bending, or lying down.

Home Remedies: *Heartburn*

Chances are, if you're suffering from heartburn, you already know it. But for an interesting test, stick out your tongue. According to traditional Chinese medicine, the tip of your tongue represents your heart. With heartburn, it is often tinged red. The middle of your tongue represents your stomach and digestive system, and it too may be very red.

So why heartburn? Your body is obviously going through great hormonal and physical changes. Traditional Chinese medicine says heartburn is linked to excessive heat in the stomach. Western medicine offers a similar theory: Hormones released during pregnancy can slow digestion and cause the valve between your stomach and esophagus to relax. Stomach acids can then seep up into your throat, causing that burning sensation. Also, as your baby grows, your uterus takes up more space, leaving less room for your stomach. Excess stomach acids have little place else to go but up!

Though there's no sure-fire heartburn preventive, here are some basic tips that might help you deter and ease your fiery symptoms:*

Avoid

- Rich, spicy, acidic, fatty, fried, and greasy foods.
- Foods containing chili powder and black, red, and hot pepper.
- Chocolate, peppermint, and spearmint.
- Oranges, grapefruit, and other acidic fruits and juices.
- Regular and decaffeinated tea and coffee, alcohol, and colas.
- Your personal trigger foods. For example—fresh bread, pastry, onions, red meat, cheese, or tomatoes.
- Overeating.
- Exercising immediately after eating.
- Bending over or lying down for at least two hours after meals.

Do

- Eat smaller meals 5–6 times a day.
- Eat slowly and chew thoroughly.
- Take a leisurely walk after meals.
- Drink smaller amounts of fluids more frequently.
- Sleep with your head elevated at least 6 inches (try adding extra pillows), or sleep upright in a comfy chair.

Try

- Eating a papaya for breakfast until symptoms improve.
- Chewing caraway, fennel, and dill seeds.
- A tablespoon of honey in a glass of warm milk.
- Drinking semi-skim milk to neutralize stomach acid.
- Fennel tea.

And if all else fails, see your caregiver—severe, continuous heartburn is a health issue that needs to be resolved.

*Always consult with your caregiver before taking antacids or natural supplements.

Babies are such a nice way to

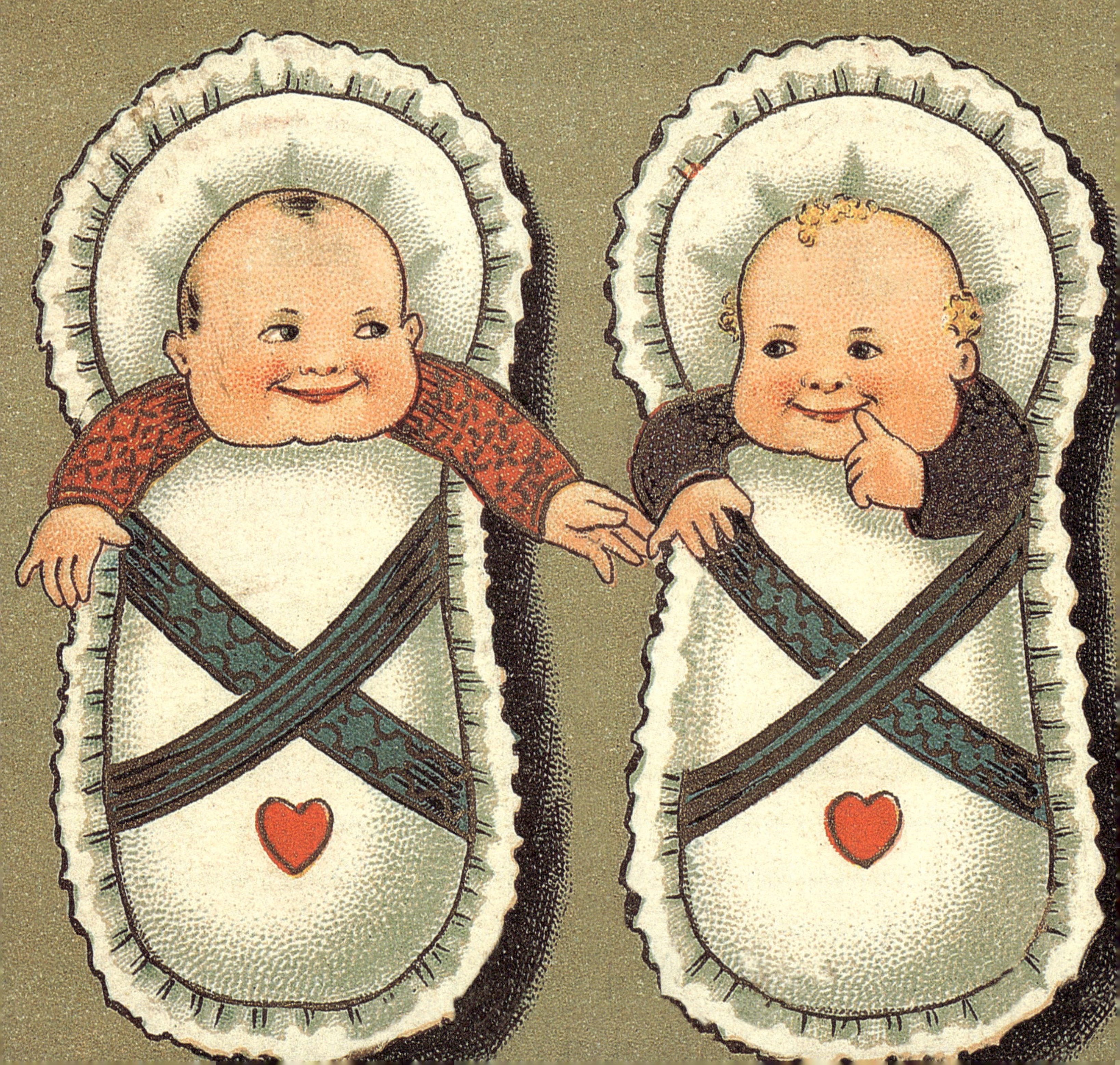

start people.–*Don Herold*

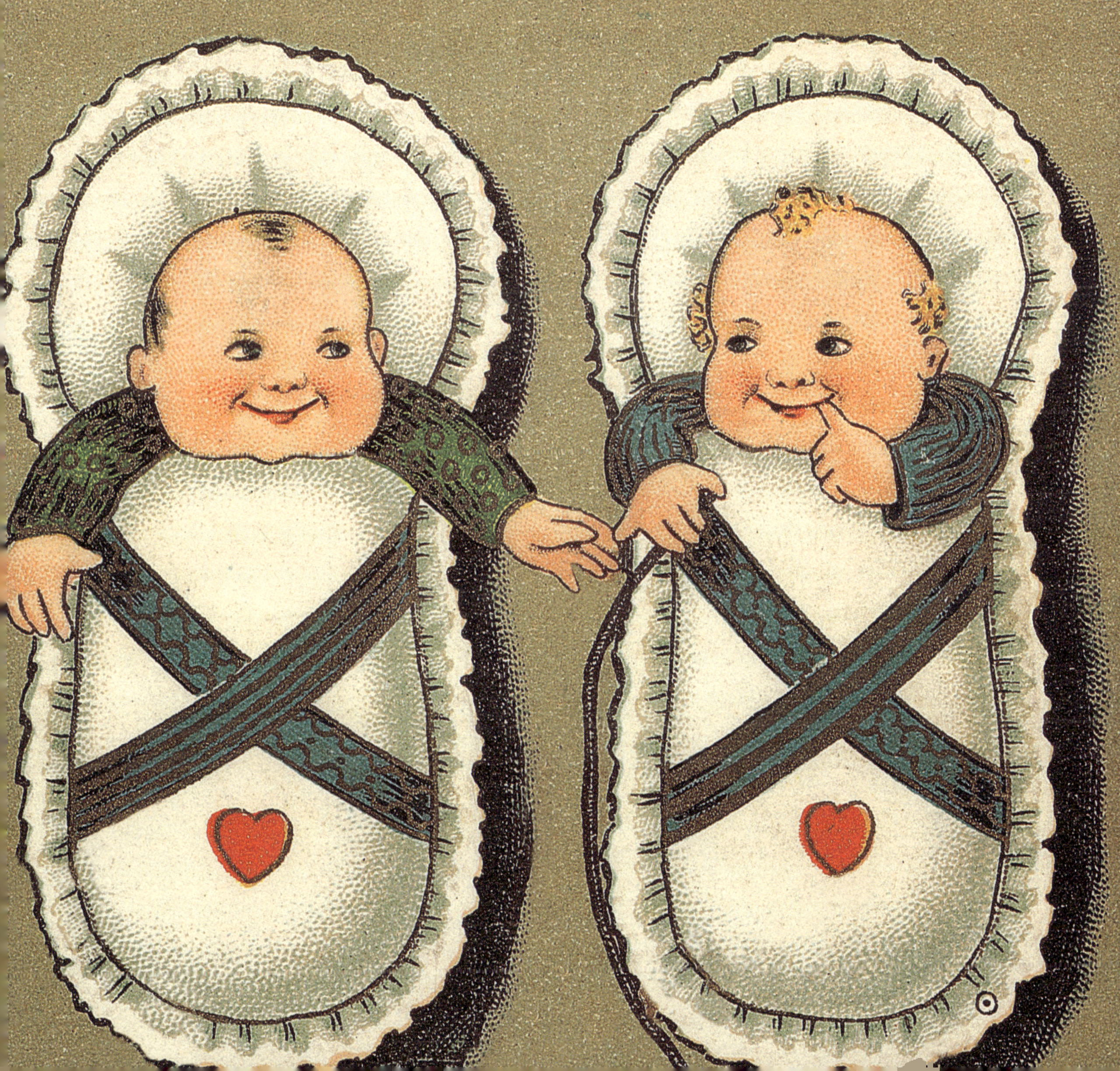

The Womb Report

- It's my third week here in the womb, and I think I feel myself thinking. Hey, that must mean my brain is starting to develop!

  Before I could feel only my mommy's heartbeat, but now there's a second one. It's small, like me. Wait—it's mine!

- *5th week*: I was just floating around today, checking out my budding limbs. My eyes have started forming, but I won't be able to use them for a while. And there are these strange floppy things forming on the side of my head. I think I'll call them "ears," because that sounds funny...hee-hee...

  Oh, and a nose has appeared on my face! I can't smell yet, but there's nothing much to smell around here anyway, except a whole lot of water. My arms look like flippers now, and my legs look like paddles, but I can't really move around. Maybe I'm becoming a fish....

- *8th week*: Hey, I can move! It seems like my brain can control how my muscles move, and I've spent the day testing them out. Never too early to start exercising, you know. And you stretch to the left! Right! Left! Right!

Some handy-dandy fingers have formed on those flippers of mine in the last few days. I can bend my arms at the elbow too, which should help with my swimming. My cool tail is starting to get very stubby, and I think it might disappear soon.

3rd month: My mouth opens whenever anything touches my face. I can't help it—it's like a reflex. I have the beginnings of vocal cords now, too, but it's going to be a while before anyone can hear me crooning. I'm also practicing breathing and sucking with my muscles. Now that my arms are almost fully formed, I spend a lot of my time gliding through the sac. Soon I'll be able to flex my hands.

And my biggest news for the month: Teeth buds! Twenty of them! One day I'll be able to eat all sorts of yummy stuff.

4th month: I can kick now, but I don't think Mommy can feel me knocking around yet, because I only weigh in at about five ounces. I can feel my heart going *thumpity-thump* harder every day, and my eyes are now pointed straight ahead instead off to the side. I guess I'm not a fish, after all....

Inspired by my new taste buds, I've started making a list of things to try. So far I've got apple pie, hot dogs, corn syrup...

❧ *5th month*: Last month I grew awfully fast, and it seems like this month will be no different. I'd guess I'm around 10 inches long now. Hmm, I wonder if Mommy can feel my kicks yet—I work hard to put every ounce of my one-pound self into each and every one. It's just my way of saying hi. Oh, and a light covering of soft hair has sprouted up all over my head and body! It's kind of neat, in a fuzzy-bear sort of way.

When I'm not busy spinning and somersaulting, I spend a good amount of time sleeping in my favorite position—with my chin resting on my chest.

❧ *6th month*: This space is getting a little tight. I must be at least a foot long! Other than that, I don't have much fat yet, so my skin looks very wrinkly. Sometimes I can hear things too, like talking and music, outside the womb—and Mommy's stomach growling.

❧ *7th month*: My eyelids have just opened for the first time. But there's not much to look at because it's so dark in here. Every now and then a little light glows through from outside Mommy's tummy and makes everything pink. I'm getting excited to see what the rest of the world looks like. On the other hand, it sure is warm and cozy in here....zzz...zzz...

❧ *8th month*: Wow! Thumbs and fingers are really fun to suck on! But I've got to be careful not to scratch myself with my newly grown fingernails. My skin is becoming more smooth and opaque, and all five of my senses are ready to work! Plus, I've got a big brain to boot. I can tell that Mommy's getting excited about how fast I'm growing. Whenever I give her a loving kick in the belly, her heart beats really fast.

- *9th month*: Wanna see me make a fist? I'm definitely getting stronger! I just passed the foot-and-a-half mark. I'm starting to get kind of chubby too, and it's making my elbows and knees dimple. It's becoming very difficult to move around in here, and most of the time I have to keep my arms crossed around my chest.

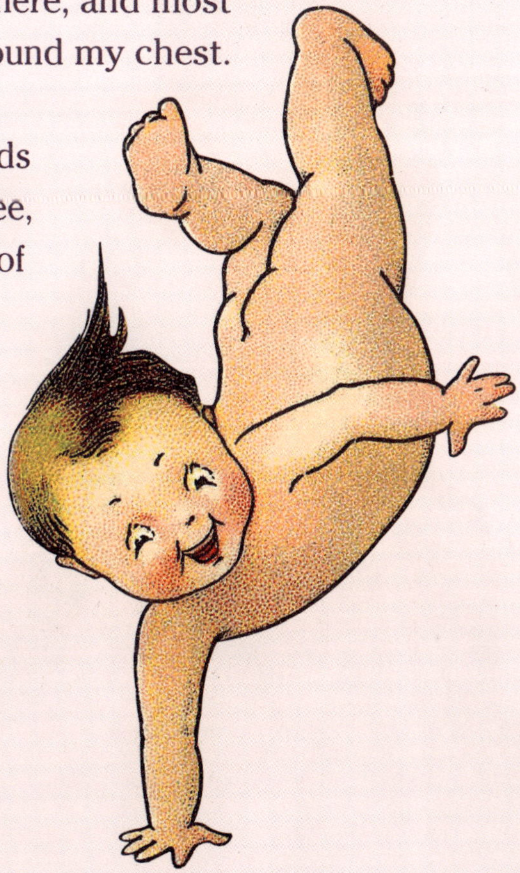

All right. Enough is enough! This big baby needs some more legroom. I think Mommy must agree, 'cause she sure is trying hard to push me out of here. You know, now that it's time, I'm having second thoughts about going. I mean, who knows what it's like out there? Maybe I'll hang on just a little longer....

Uh-oh, I'm losing my grip....

Wow! This is some ride!

Yippee! Look out world
—HERE COMES BABY!

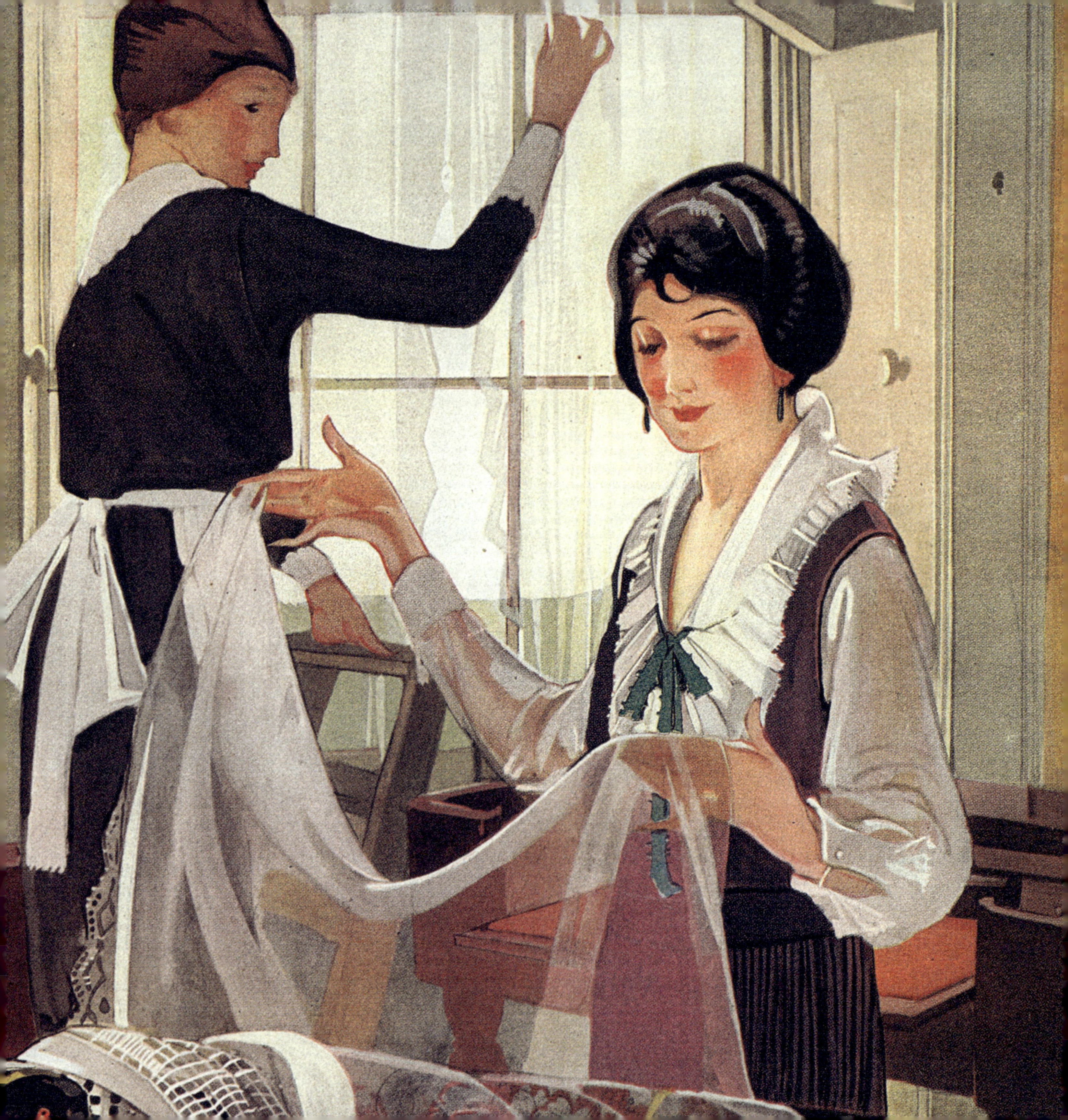

Special Tips

Decorating the nursery is a great way to personally welcome your child into his new home and satisfy those irresistible maternal nesting urges all at once. You want baby's room to be the most nurturing and beautiful haven possible. This is the space where your little one will spend most of his early days sleeping, eating, and observing his world. There are so many ways to make the nursery a special, soothing, and stimulating environment. Here are just a few ideas to inspire you.

A Crib with a View

Remember, your baby will sleep through much of her early life. That means she'll spend many hours in her crib examining the ceiling above. So give her something to look at! Hang mobiles or shiny crystals and paint pictures on the ceiling. Place the crib in the center of the room and give baby a panoramic view. Nothing delights an infant more than seeing her reflection. Secure a mirror to a wall near the crib and watch baby amuse herself for hours.

Sound Ideas

Sound is very important in the nursery. The music you listened to while you were expecting can comfort a cranky infant. The soft soothing trickle of a small water fountain or the tinkling of wind chimes also can relax baby (and mother, too.)

Clever Changing Table

Convert the top of a desk or chest of drawers into a changing table by adding a simple 3- to 4-inch-thick foam mat. Cut the foam 8 inches narrower than the desktop or chest. Trim a nonskid rug pad to the same size as the foam. Glue the pad to the bottom of the foam. Cover the top of the foam with waterproof sheeting. Wrap the top and sides of the foam neatly with a baby bath towel, which can be changed often. Presto! You've got a brand-new changing table!

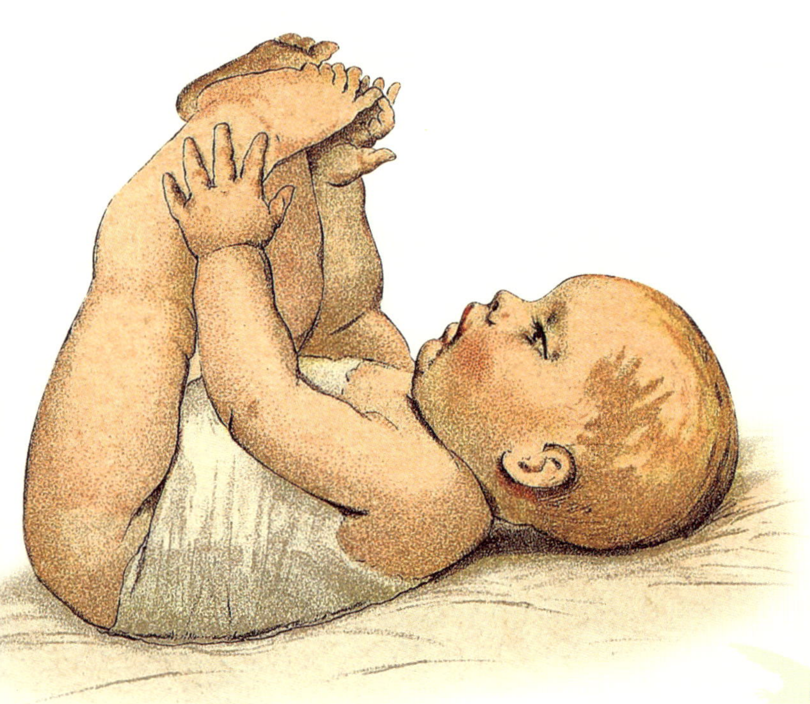

Antique Baby Dresser

An old armoire makes a great baby dresser. Add a fresh coat of white paint and install two closet rods (available at your local hardware store) in the top cupboard for hanging little clothes. Stack diapers on the bottom shelf.

Darling Details

After the basics (crib, drawers, rocker and pillow, lamp) indulge in details and follow a theme. Noah's Ark or a barnyard or zoo scene works well for an animal-loving family. Stencil an animal border, paint animal footprints on the floor, or hang stuffed-animal birds from the ceiling! Consider a nature motif with clouds on the ceiling, a butterfly mobile, and a painted family tree on the wall (see following pages for nature theme how-to.) Another unique idea: Frame your favorite children's book illustrations or paste them to the wall to make a very special border.

Nifty Thrifties

You don't have to spend a lot to be creative. Loads of decorative ideas can be implemented using what you already have. When seeking inspiration: Recycle! Save the ribbons from shower gifts to make a bright mobile, and the wrapping paper to line baby's drawers and shelves. Or make a collage on baby's closet door using all of the congratulatory messages and gift cards you've received, and shower invitations and birth announcements you've sent out.

Precious Laundry Bag

A simple and sweet laundry bag can be made with an "orphan" vintage pillowcase. Simply make two small holes in the hem of the case on either side of the seam. Attach a large safety pin to the end of one yard of 1-inch-wide grosgrain ribbon. Use the pin to manipulate the ribbon in one hole, through the hem, and out the other hole, creating a drawstring. Tie the ends of the ribbon together and hang the decorative bag on a doorknob or use to line a plastic pail for baby's laundry.

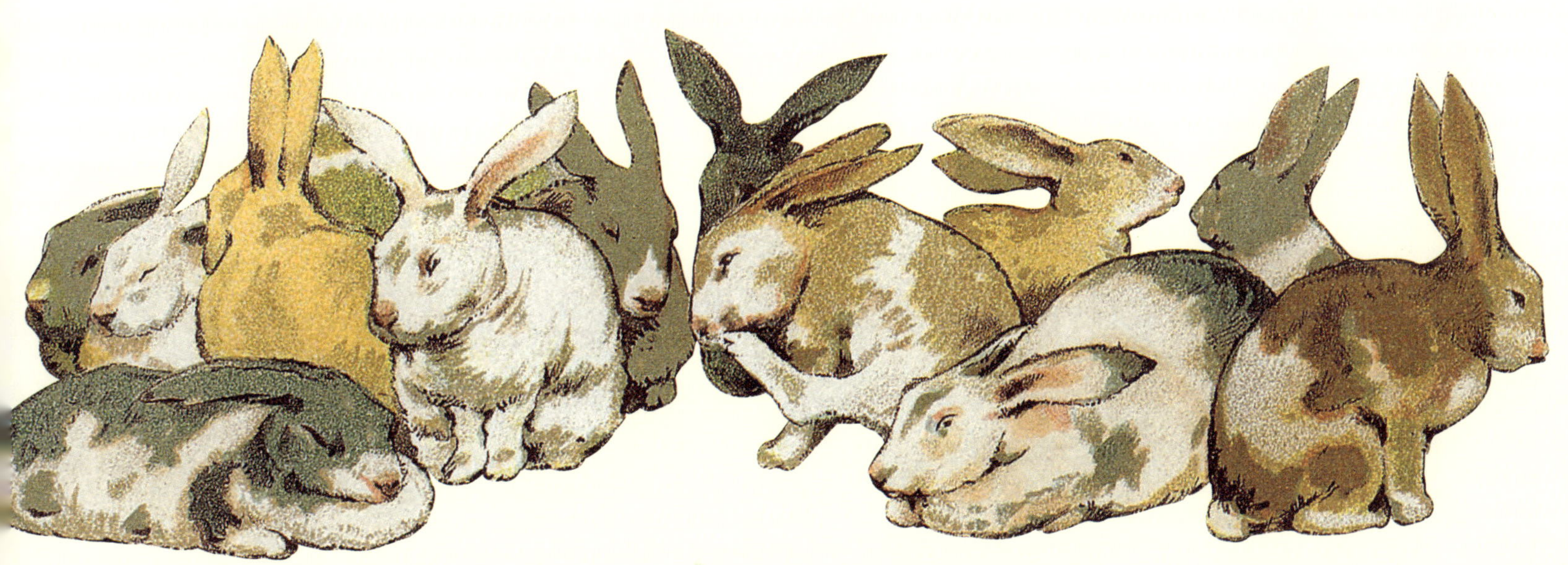

Sky Ceiling

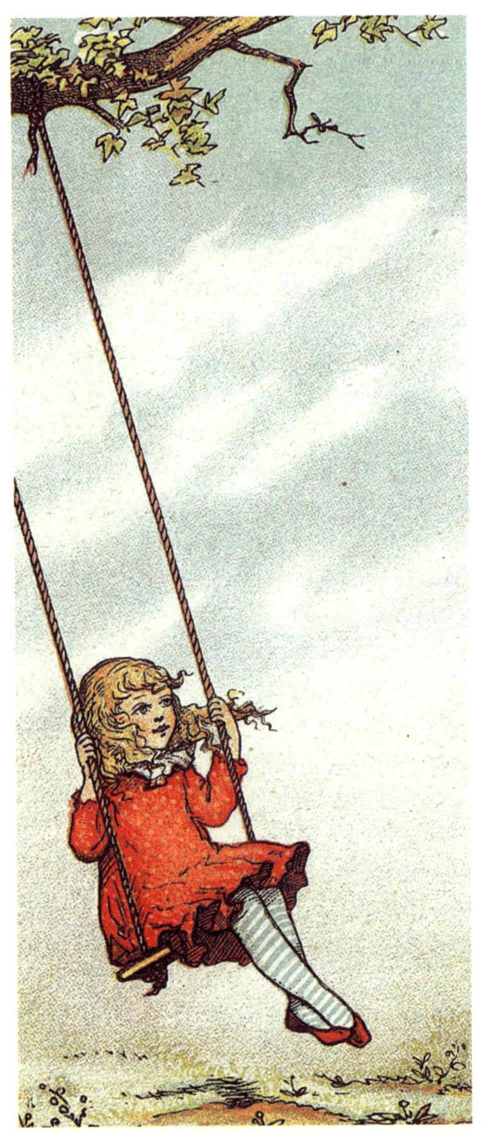

Bring the outside world inside your baby's nursery with a hand-painted sky ceiling. Recreate the comforting feeling of a warm spring afternoon as the clouds roll lazily overhead. It's easy to do, even if you're not particularly crafty! This view from the crib is certain to delight baby for years. As an added effect, decorate the ceiling with glow-in-the-dark stars and watch your nursery go from daytime to nighttime with a flick of a switch. This is also a neat decorating idea for a child's playroom.

You will need:

Latex interior wall paint in your favorite light blue (1 gal. = 350–400 sq. ft. per coat)

1 pint white latex interior wall paint

Large paintbrush or roller and tray

1 or 2 large natural sea sponges, slightly damp

Optional: acrylic craft/artists' paint

1. Prepare the ceiling as directed on the paint can and apply one to two coats (as necessary) of light blue paint. You may want to create a vaulted ceiling effect by extending the color down the walls several inches, making a border. Allow paint to fully dry after each coat.

2. Pour a little of the white paint into a disposable pie tin or plastic plate. Thin with an equal amount of water, adding a little at a time, mixing well.

3. To create clouds, lightly dip the damp sponge into the watered-down paint. Start from the center of each cloud and work outward in circles, repeatedly dabbing the sponge to apply an almost transparent white layer of paint in cloud shapes. Be creative. Vary the sizes and shapes of your clouds.

4. When you finish the first cloud layer, let it dry, and then sponge each cloud lightly again with a mixture of paint and half the amount of water, *allowing patches of the first layer to show through*, especially around the edges of your clouds.

5. Apply a third layer sparingly, highlighting your clouds with white undiluted paint, again allowing the first two layers to show through here and there.

6. If you're feeling especially creative, add a few passing birds or butterflies using the acrylic craft/artists' paint.

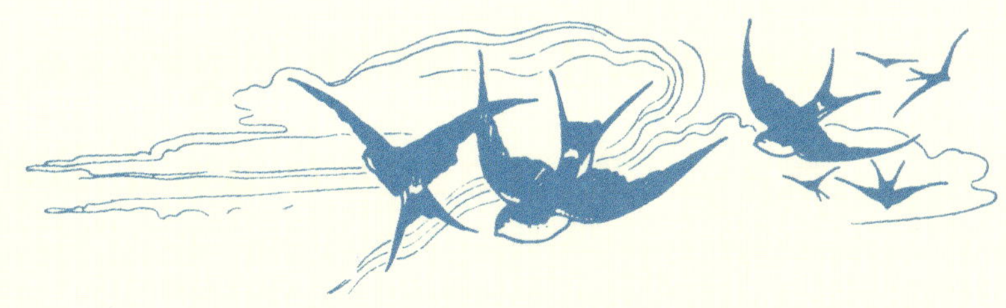

Can I regard my pregnancy as anything but one long festival?... I especially remember how at odd hours sleep overwhelmed me and how I was seized again, as in my infancy, by the need to sleep on the ground, on the grass, on the sun-warmed hay. A unique and healthy craving.

–Colette

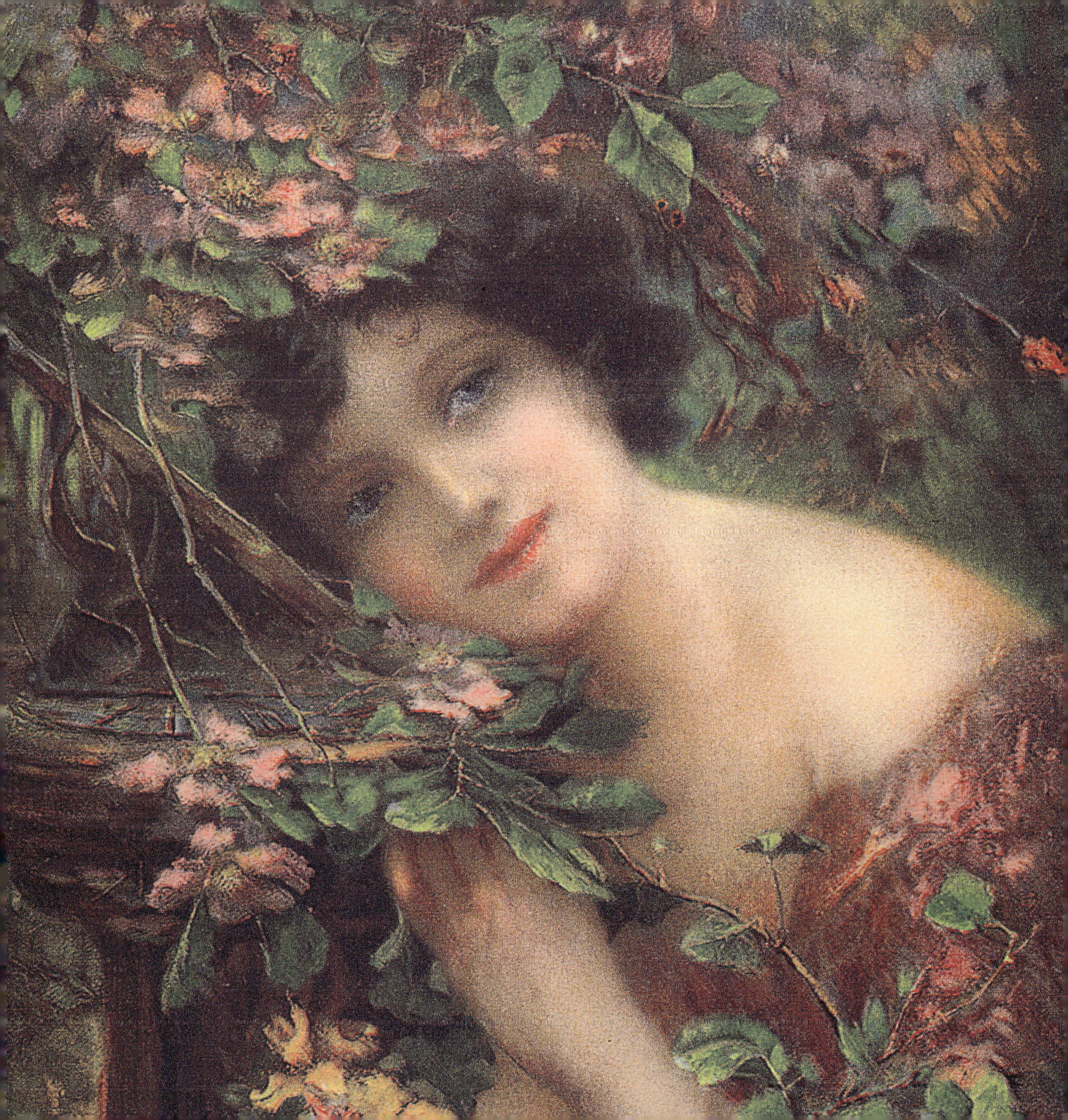

Crazy Cravings

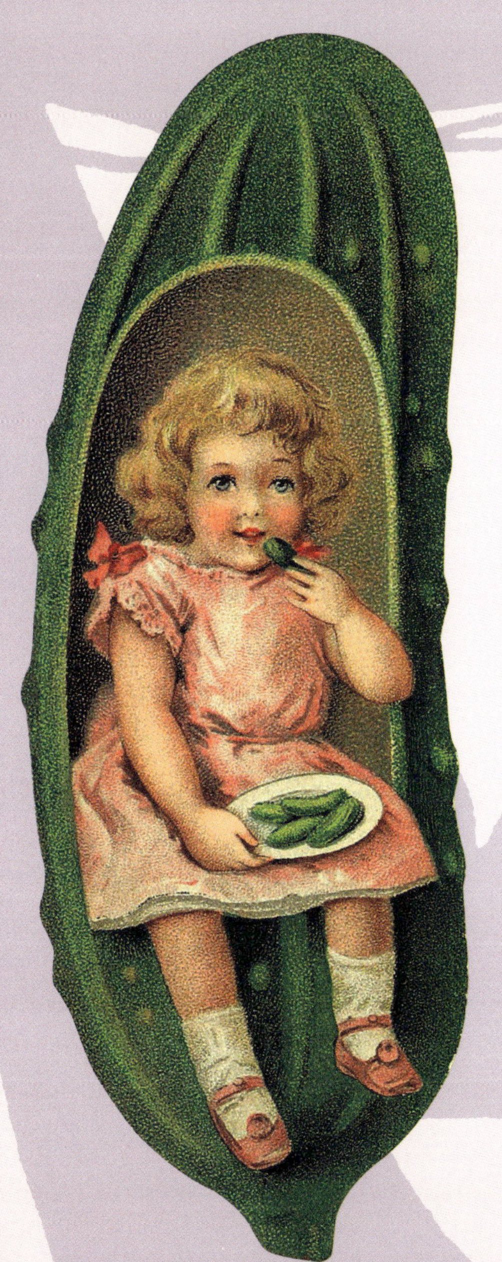

Are you constantly running to the store for more chocolate mint ice cream? Is your appetite for greasy fries impossible to curb? Well, you're not alone. Statistically speaking, more than two-thirds of all women report at least one strong food craving during pregnancy. Shifting hormones, an altered sense of taste and smell, and changes in your nutritional requirements are to blame. Some women have an insatiable desire for sweets, particularly chocolate. Others crave salty foods, like olives, pickles, and potato chips. But are all cravings bad?

Most healthcare professionals agree that a yearning for a particular food is only bad insomuch as it causes an imbalance in your diet. So, try to satisfy your yens with a variety of foods, and avoid the junk-food cravings by finding substitutes. Next time the salt bug bites, pass on the bottomless bag of fatty potato chips. Reach instead for baked chips or soft pretzels. Satisfy your passion for a hot-fudge sundae or chocolate shake with a nonfat frozen yoghurt or smoothie. And if you crave oranges, nectarines, broccoli, and collard greens, consider yourself lucky and, by all means, indulge!

THE PROVERBIAL PICKLES AND ICE CREAM

Bizarre culinary combinations abound during pregnancy. And, although we don't know any mothers who'd kill for pickles dipped in Rocky Road, here's what some had to say about their cravings:

"During my first trimester, I craved the foods of my childhood. When I was little my mom would make grilled-cheese sandwiches and tomato soup, tuna melts, cottage cheese and fruit (in sweet syrup, of course), and macaroni and cheese with hot dogs—very glamorous foods, all. But that wasn't even the worst of it. My cravings for the sweets of my youth also returned in full force. Try reigning in an obsession for Necco wafers, Sweet Tarts, and Red Vines. I'm just lucky that Fun Dip is so hard to find these days."

"When I was pregnant with my daughter, I longed for mushrooms. This fact astonished me, as I had never been a mushroom enthusiast—in truth, I was quite the opposite. Sure enough, as soon as she was born, my aversion returned."

"With each of my pregnancies, I have experienced an overwhelming desire for anything orange—carrots, yams, and sweet potatoes; peaches, papaya, and cantaloupe; pumpkin pie, butterscotch pudding, and orange sherbet. And I can't leave out the goldfish crackers! If it was orange...I was eating it."

"Apples! That's all I wanted, for breakfast, lunch, and dinner."

So, the next time you wake up at two in the morning with a yen for yams and Jell-O, don't feel guilty. Just remember, it comes with the territory.

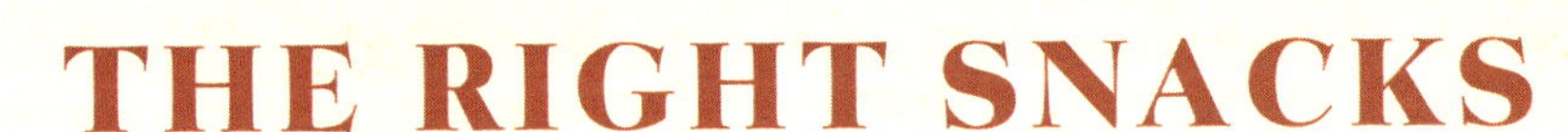

THE RIGHT SNACKS

Finding it harder to pack a full meal into your ever-shrinking stomach? Does your hunger strike more frequently these days? Try eating smaller meals more often. In truth, it is a healthier way to live—as long as you're making sound food choices. So, next time you have a snack attack, reach for something healthy. Bite down on a banana or whole-wheat crackers and some low-fat string cheese. Munch on an apple and some yoghurt, half a peanut butter and jelly (preferably whole-fruit spread) sandwich and a pear, edamame (green soy beans in the pod), low- or nonfat cottage cheese and fruit, dried fruits and nuts, or a bowl of cereal and milk. Or try one of our recipes.

HOMEMADE GRANOLA

(Benefits: This low-fat, low-sugar treat provides a lasting energy boost.)

Ingredients

1 1/2 cups rolled oats
1/4 cup chopped almonds
2 tablespoons sugar
1 1/2 tablespoons ground cinnamon
Optional: dried cherries, cranberries, or apricots; raisins; wheat germ; and sunflower or pumpkin seeds.

1. Preheat oven to 350 degrees.
2. Combine all ingredients in a medium bowl and mix well. Spread the mixture on a baking sheet or in a shallow pan.
3. Bake for 25 to 30 minutes, or until light brown, stirring frequently. Let cool completely and then store in an airtight container. Granola should keep for at least a week.
4. Serve with fruit, yoghurt, or as a topping for ice cream or frozen yoghurt.

Makes 2 cups.

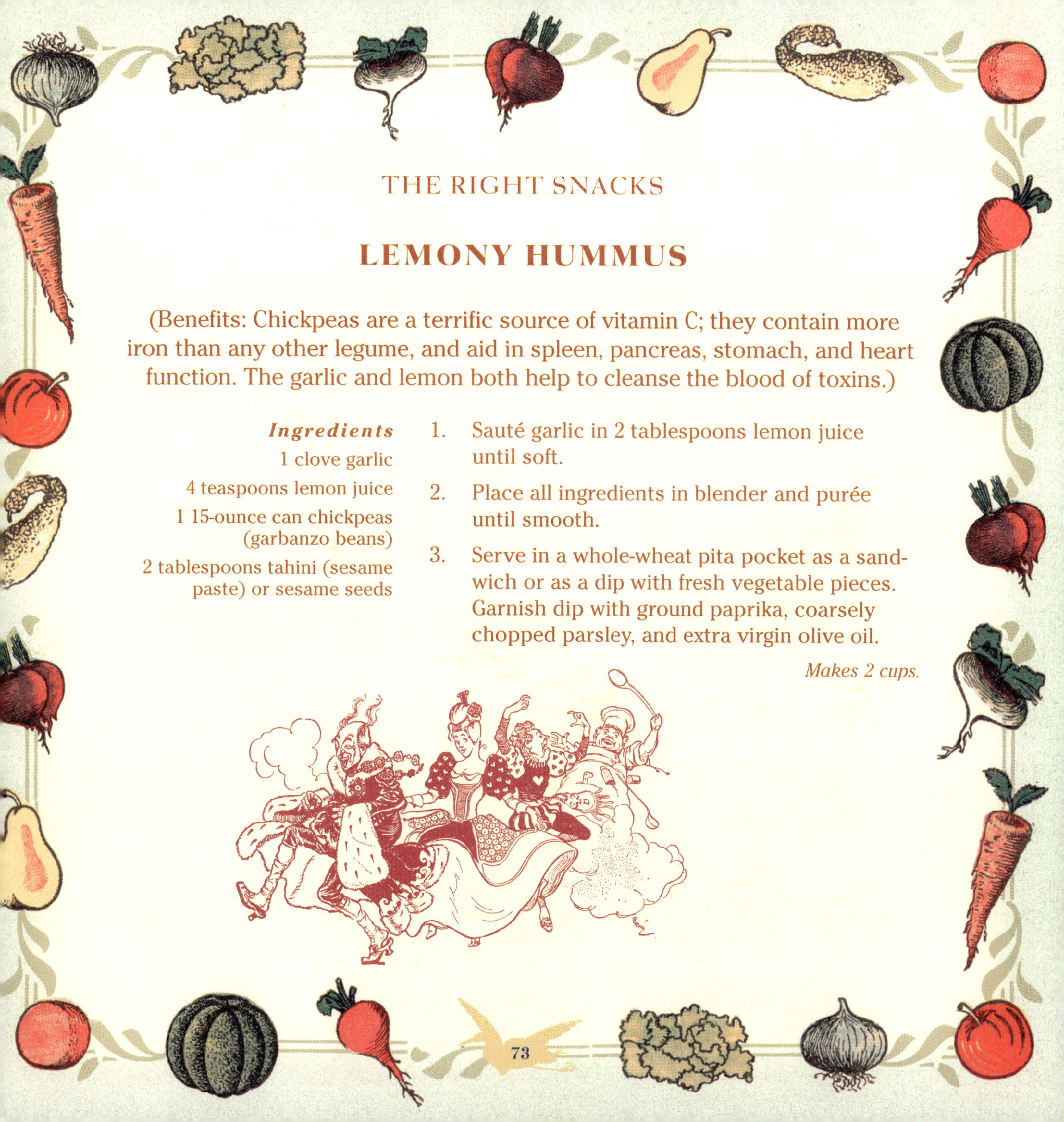

LEMONY HUMMUS

(Benefits: Chickpeas are a terrific source of vitamin C; they contain more iron than any other legume, and aid in spleen, pancreas, stomach, and heart function. The garlic and lemon both help to cleanse the blood of toxins.)

Ingredients

1 clove garlic

4 teaspoons lemon juice

1 15-ounce can chickpeas (garbanzo beans)

2 tablespoons tahini (sesame paste) or sesame seeds

1. Sauté garlic in 2 tablespoons lemon juice until soft.
2. Place all ingredients in blender and purée until smooth.
3. Serve in a whole-wheat pita pocket as a sandwich or as a dip with fresh vegetable pieces. Garnish dip with ground paprika, coarsely chopped parsley, and extra virgin olive oil.

Makes 2 cups.

SIMPLE QUESADILLA

(Benefits: With the right fillings, this tasty snack doubles as a well-balanced mini-meal.)

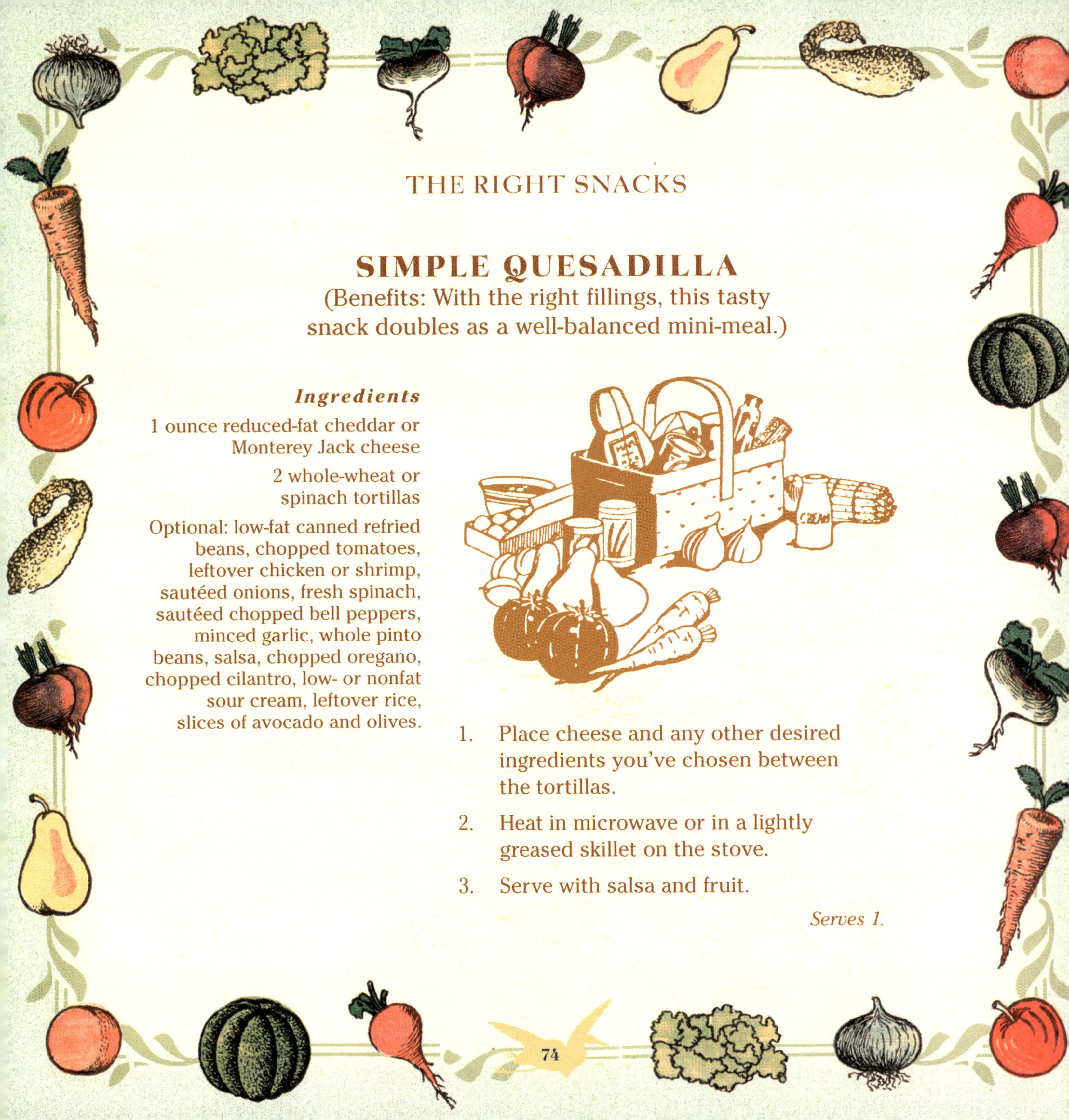

Ingredients

1 ounce reduced-fat cheddar or Monterey Jack cheese

2 whole-wheat or spinach tortillas

Optional: low-fat canned refried beans, chopped tomatoes, leftover chicken or shrimp, sautéed onions, fresh spinach, sautéed chopped bell peppers, minced garlic, whole pinto beans, salsa, chopped oregano, chopped cilantro, low- or nonfat sour cream, leftover rice, slices of avocado and olives.

1. Place cheese and any other desired ingredients you've chosen between the tortillas.
2. Heat in microwave or in a lightly greased skillet on the stove.
3. Serve with salsa and fruit.

Serves 1.

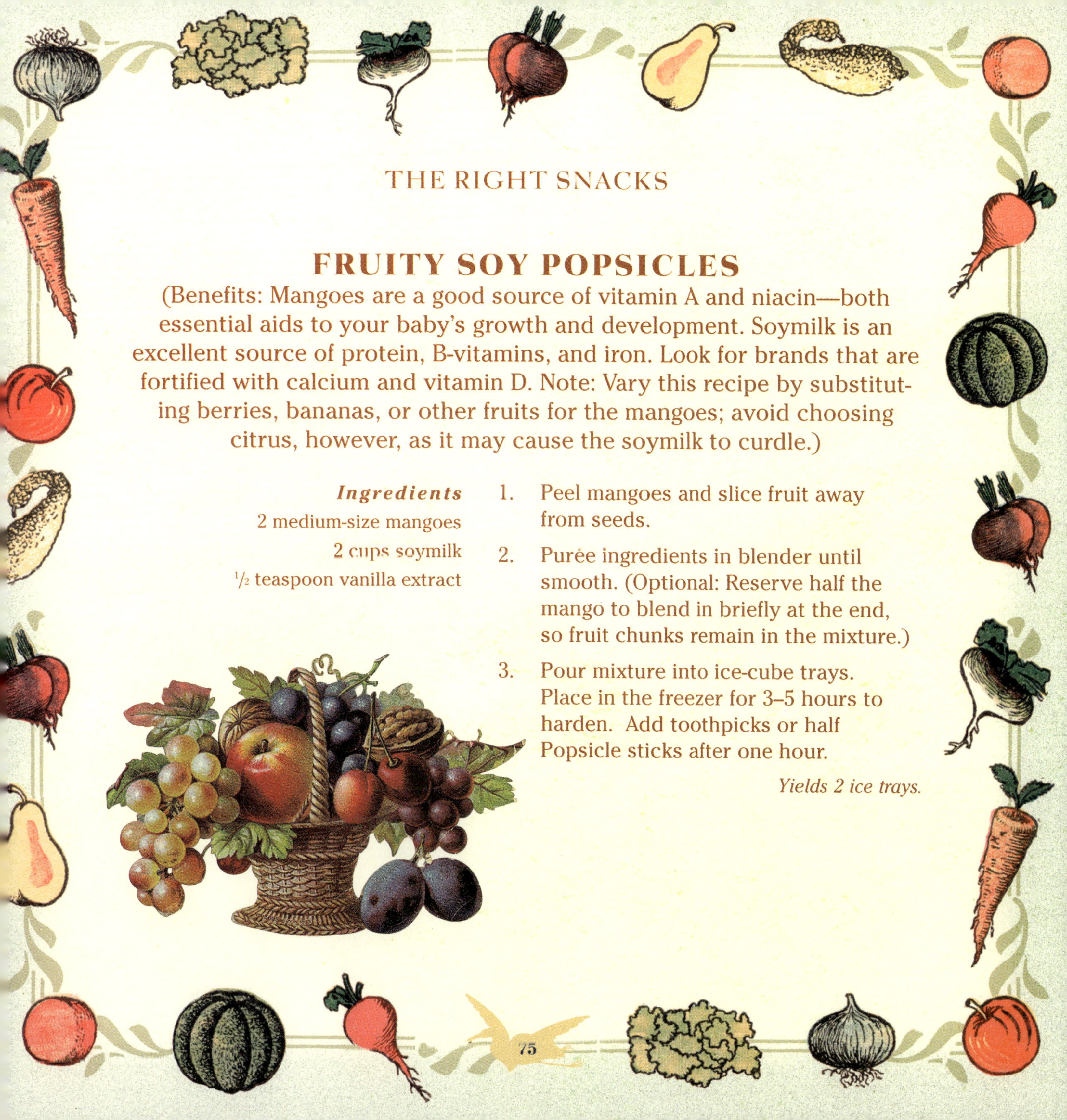

FRUITY SOY POPSICLES

(Benefits: Mangoes are a good source of vitamin A and niacin—both essential aids to your baby's growth and development. Soymilk is an excellent source of protein, B-vitamins, and iron. Look for brands that are fortified with calcium and vitamin D. Note: Vary this recipe by substituting berries, bananas, or other fruits for the mangoes; avoid choosing citrus, however, as it may cause the soymilk to curdle.)

Ingredients

2 medium-size mangoes

2 cups soymilk

½ teaspoon vanilla extract

1. Peel mangoes and slice fruit away from seeds.
2. Purée ingredients in blender until smooth. (Optional: Reserve half the mango to blend in briefly at the end, so fruit chunks remain in the mixture.)
3. Pour mixture into ice-cube trays. Place in the freezer for 3–5 hours to harden. Add toothpicks or half Popsicle sticks after one hour.

Yields 2 ice trays.

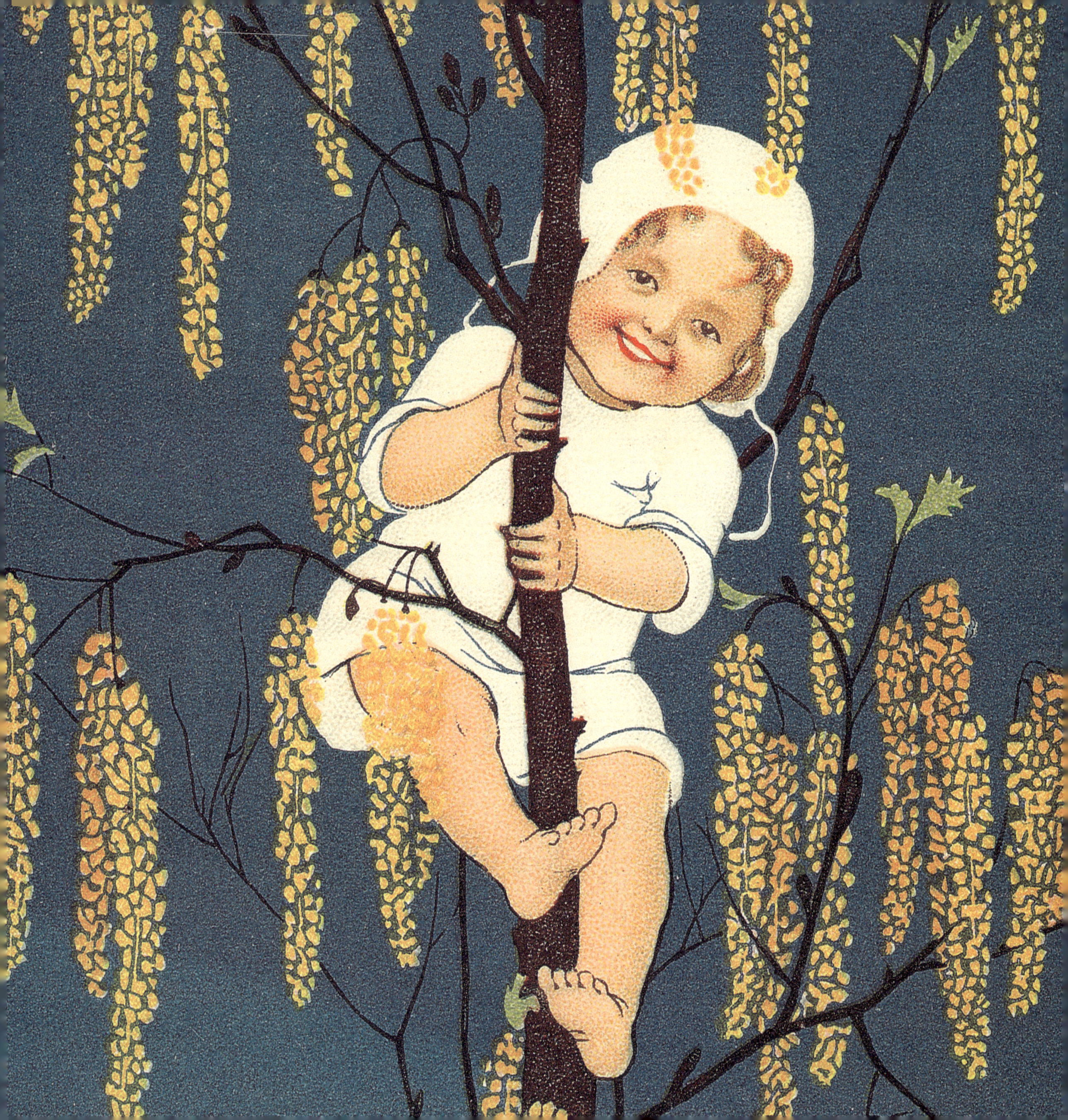

The rules for parents are but three...Love, Limit, and Let them be.

–Elaine M. Ward

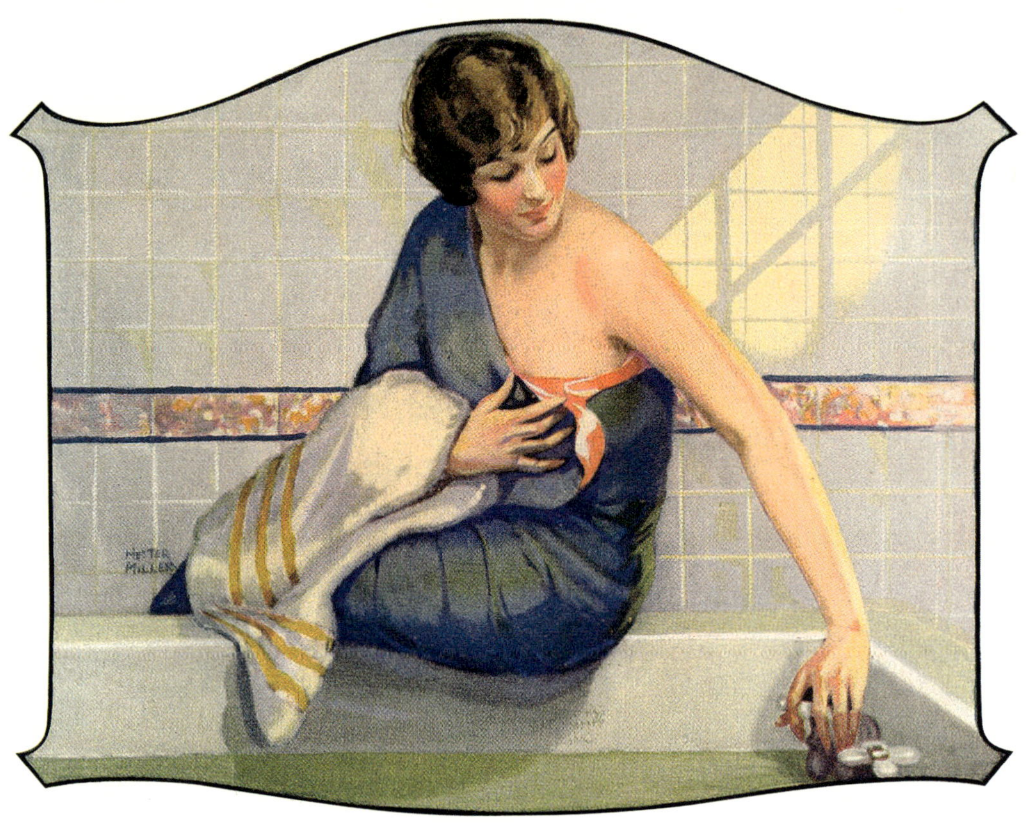

SPA DAY

Pregnancy can be a stressful time. You can even get stressed worrying about stress! Eating well, getting your rest, exercising, and stretching all help keep you balanced. But sometimes you need a little extra pampering. So, go ahead. Put your feet up. Walk in the fresh air. Read a book. Watch an old movie. Better yet, take a "spa day" for yourself, or at least a spa hour. Here are some suggestions:

Soothing Soaks

What could be better than slipping into a tub of warm water? A cozy bath can do wonders for lack of energy, sore muscles, insomnia, and the strain your increasing girth places on your body. And these are just the physical benefits!

1. Start by turning your bathroom into a sanctuary. Light some candles. Play restful music. Prop up your bath pillow. Get a tall glass of ice water with lemon to keep yourself hydrated.

2. Then draw your bath...but not too hot (high temperatures are dangerous during pregnancy).

3. Add rose petals to uplift your mood or lemon slices to refresh and stimulate your senses. Use a few drops of essential oils—bergamot, chamomile, or lavender—to help you relax. (Caution: The oils we recommend are safe to use, but certain essential oils are contraindicated during pregnancy. Please check with your healthcare provider before experimenting.)

4. Now, step in. Lie back, close your eyes, and release yourself from the stresses of the day. Practice the slow breathing and relaxation techniques you have been learning in your childbirth classes. Then look at your belly rising above the water. Enjoy its roundness. Watch the water ripple as your baby kicks....

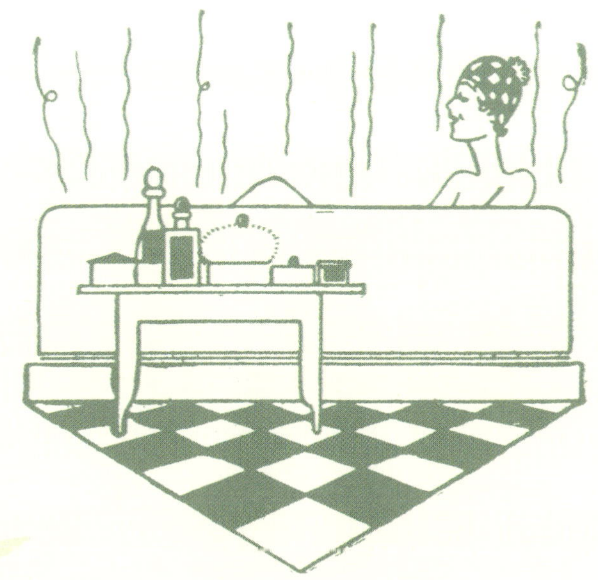

The Ultimate Facial

A soothing facial includes four key factors: steaming, cleaning, toning, and moisturizing. *Note*: Our cleanser doubles as an exfoliant.

STEAM: Soak a hand towel in a bowl of warm chamomile tea. Wrap the towel on your face and neck and leave it until cool. Repeat if desired. This process will open up pores for deeper cleansing. (Reserve some tea for the next step.)

CLEANSE & EXFOLIATE: Apply our Chamomile and Oats Cleanser/Exfoliant (see recipe below) in upward circular motions to stimulate skin and work out dirt and oil. Rinse thoroughly with warm water and pat face dry.

TONE: Soak a cotton ball with Rosewater Toner (see recipe on next page.) Gently pat the toner all over your face and neck. Don't rub. Leave to dry naturally.

MOISTURIZE: While your skin is still damp from the toner, apply a generous amount of 100 percent aloe vera gel to your face and neck. Let it soak in for 2–3 minutes before removing any excess gel with a soft tissue. For very dry spots, use small drops of pure Vitamin E.

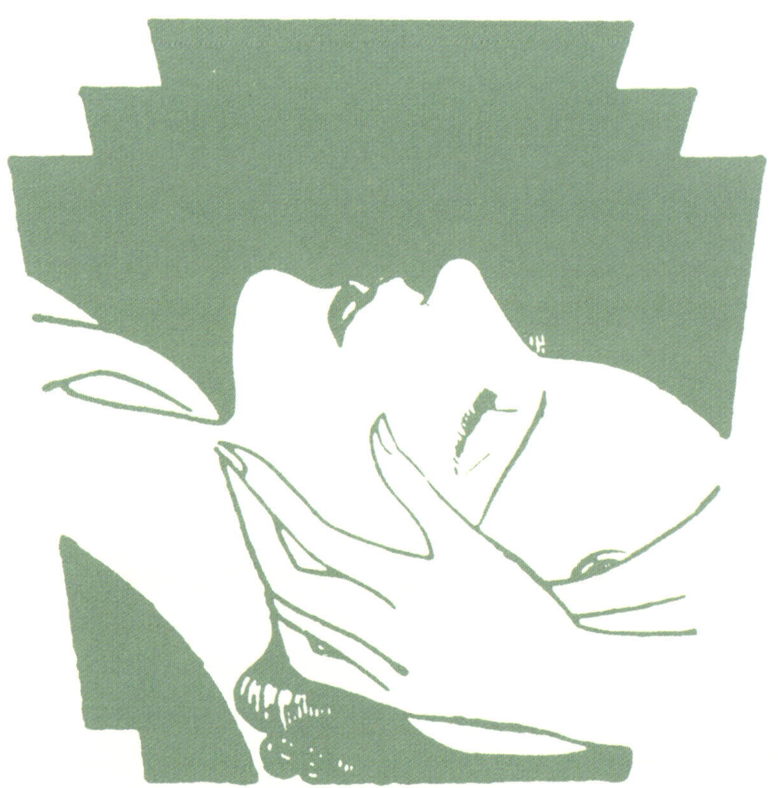

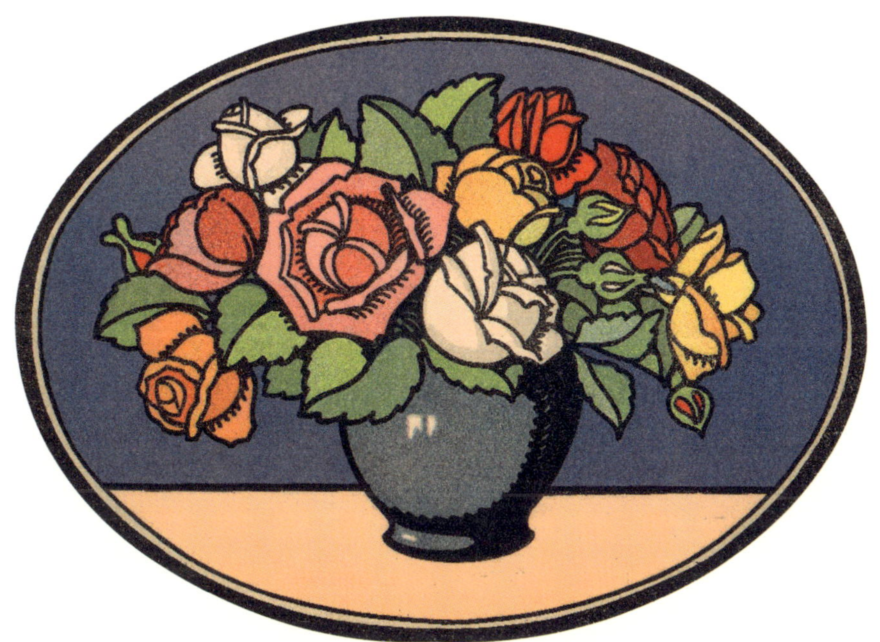

Recipes:

Chamomile and Oatmeal Cleanser/Exfoliant

2 tablespoons brewed chamomile tea (reserved from STEAM step)

1 tablespoon finely ground oats

1 tablespoon finely ground almonds

1 teaspoon honey

1 tablespoon 100% aloe vera gel

Combine all ingredients in a bowl and stir until well mixed.

Rosewater Toner

3 large handfuls fresh red rose petals

1 quart distilled water

1 sterile storage bottle

1. Place rose petals in a small saucepan.
2. Pour distilled water over petals and simmer on low heat until half the water is absorbed.
3. Allow the water to cool before discarding the petals. Pour the rosewater into the sterile storage bottle.

Home Remedies: Aches & Pains

All these changes—some are wondrous, but some are a pain in the neck! Or is it your back? Actually it's more of a leg cramp....Well, it's no secret that as your baby grows and your body prepares for delivery, you'll experience some brand-new aches and pains. The good news is that with extra attention and care, you can work to prevent or assuage many of your pangs.

Oh, My Aching Back

Most pregnant women experience backaches, especially during the last trimester. As your pregnancy progresses, the increasing weight of your baby changes your center of gravity. To maintain balance, you may tend to arch your neck, pull back your shoulders, and push your belly forward. Unfortunately, these adjustments can greatly strain your back muscles. In addition, your body produces pregnancy hormones that start softening up ligaments, loosening up the spine and pelvis and preparing for the birth of the baby. Your destabilized pelvis can add to lower back strain.

So read through our tips, consider your changing body, and give some support to your poor aching back. And if your pain is continuous, severe, or runs down your leg toward your foot, be sure to consult your caregiver—a slipped disc can be serious business!

- Practice good posture by holding your spine straight when walking or standing. Try not to slouch and don't stand for too long. When standing, relieve stress by standing on a cushioned mat or with one foot up on a stool.
- When seated, sit with your back straight, your buttocks all the way to the back of the chair, and, if possible, your legs slightly elevated. Use chair arms to help you get up and avoid unsupportive, overly-cushioned, or backless chairs.
- Resist the urge to cross your legs while sitting. It can cause circulation troubles and exacerbate back problems by overly tilting your pelvis. Believe it or not, sitting can strain your back more than almost any other activity. Don't sit for too long—every 30 minutes, get up and stretch or take a short walk.
- Avoid bending forward, reaching high over your head, or making sudden, jerky movements.
- Learn to lift properly. Squat down, bending your knees and hips and keeping your back vertical. Grasp the item, close to your body, and slowly stand, lifting with your leg muscles, never bending at your waist. Avoid picking up heavy items, especially after your first trimester, and don't be shy about asking for help.
- Wear comfortable, low-heeled shoes that offer good support. Ask your caregiver or shoe salesperson about supportive inserts or shoes designed for extra comfort.
- Sleep on a firm, quality mattress with pillows supporting your legs and back. If your mattress is too soft, try placing a board under it. In the morning, slide your legs over the side of the bed and push yourself up into a sitting position.
- Relieve aching muscles with a warm bath in the morning and at night.
- Try to keep your weight within the recommended range to help ease the load on your back.
- Talk to your caregiver about supporting your back with a pregnancy girdle or a crisscross belly-support sling.

Ye-ouch—Charley Horse!

If you've ever had a cramp, or "charley horse," you know it's a sharply painful muscle spasm and it's certainly no fun. Cramps during pregnancy are often triggered by fatigue, changes in circulation, the additional weight you're carrying, or holding your body in a tense, awkward position. Leg and foot cramps are very common, especially at night during your last trimester, when you're trying to get some much-needed shuteye. And though the painful spasms usually last for only a moment, the affected muscle may continue to ache for some time after.

Thankfully, cramps often can be prevented or quickly soothed; if they continuously plague you, though, be sure to talk to your caregiver about solutions. Infrequently, a cramp may signify a blood clot, which is a serious medical condition.

Here are some suggestions to keep that mean charley horse at bay:

- If you elect to exercise during your pregnancy, always do a thorough warm-up and stretch for at least 15 minutes beforehand.
- Make sure to drink plenty of water and other fluids throughout the day.
- Try wearing support hose.
- Be sure to take breaks during the day, resting with your feet elevated.

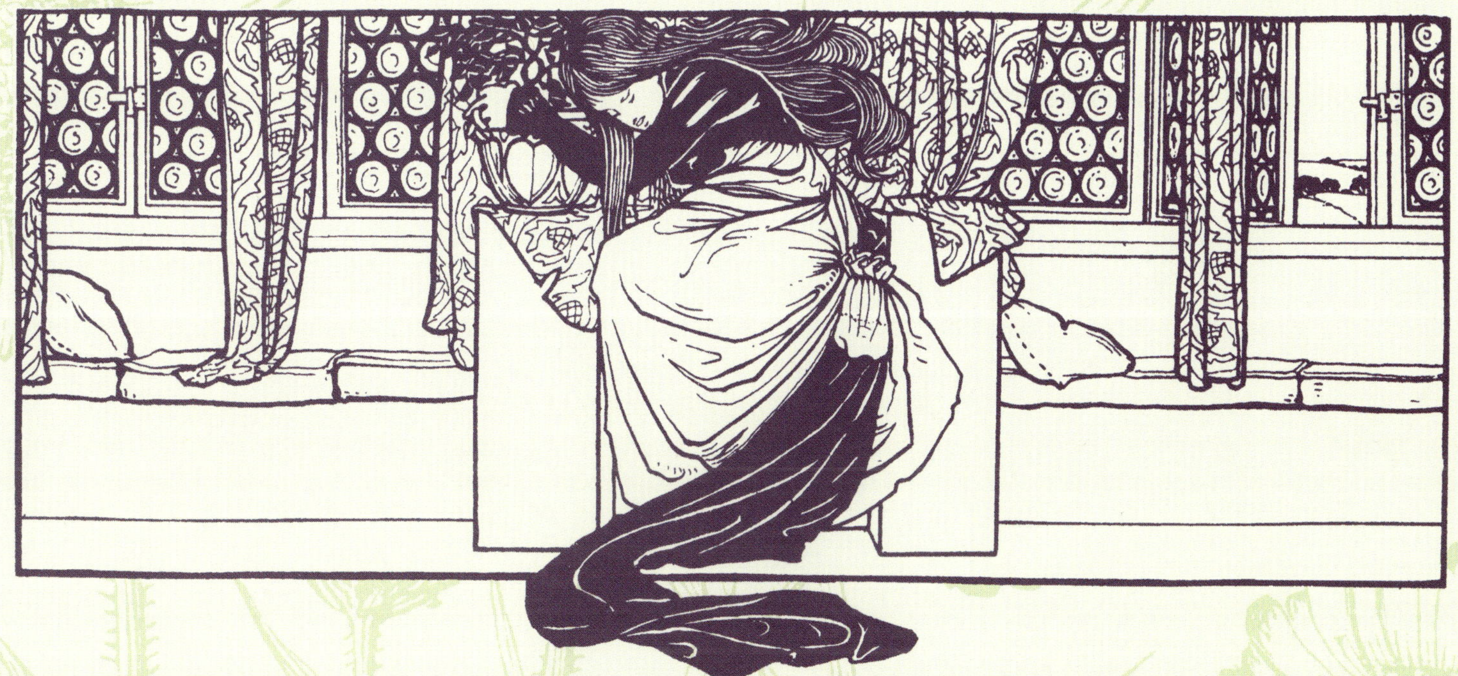

But if a charley horse gives you a good kick:

- Firmly massage the cramping muscle. Gently stretch your calf by flexing your foot, bringing your toes toward your face and pushing your heels down.
- For a more strenuous stretch, stand a half foot back from the wall or a sturdy chair. Put your hands on the wall or grip the back of the chair and slowly slide the cramping leg back, keeping your leg straight and your heel on the floor. Bend your other knee as you slide. Slide your leg back in and repeat as necessary.
- Flexing your feet and stretching your calves before bed may help prevent nighttime cramps.
- Use a warm compress to enhance your circulation and relieve the cramp.
- Some say that standing on a cold floor can help ease cramping.

Kegel Exercises

What are they? What is the point? How do I do them? Kegel exercises are a muscle-group isolation technique that serves to tighten the pelvic floor muscles that support the urethra, bladder, uterus, and rectum. Strengthening the pelvic floor muscles will help you:

- maintain better bladder control during and after pregnancy
- condition your body for an easier childbirth (fewer tears in the perineum)
- improve sex for you and your partner during pregnancy and after delivery

The most important step in learning how to perform a Kegel is to identify the target muscles. Here is one simple way to do this. Contract your pelvic muscles as you would to stop the flow of urine. Repeat this a few times until you get the feel of isolating the correct muscle group. To practice a Kegel, contract the muscles for a count of 10–20 seconds, and then release for another few seconds. Repeat ten to twenty times. It is recommended that you perform the exercise two to three times a day. You can practice Kegels anywhere, anytime—no one will know but you!

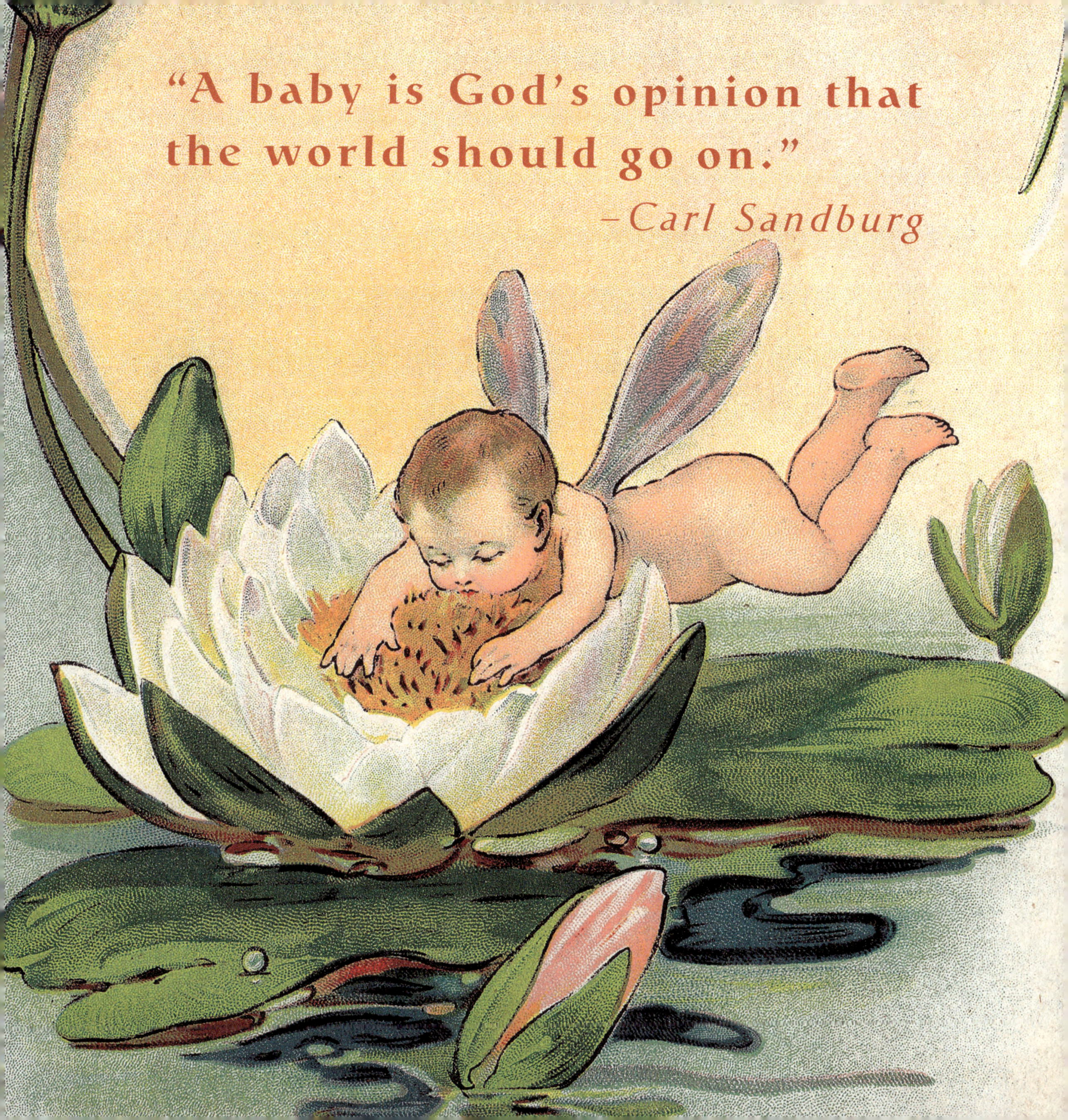
"A baby is God's opinion that the world should go on."
–Carl Sandburg

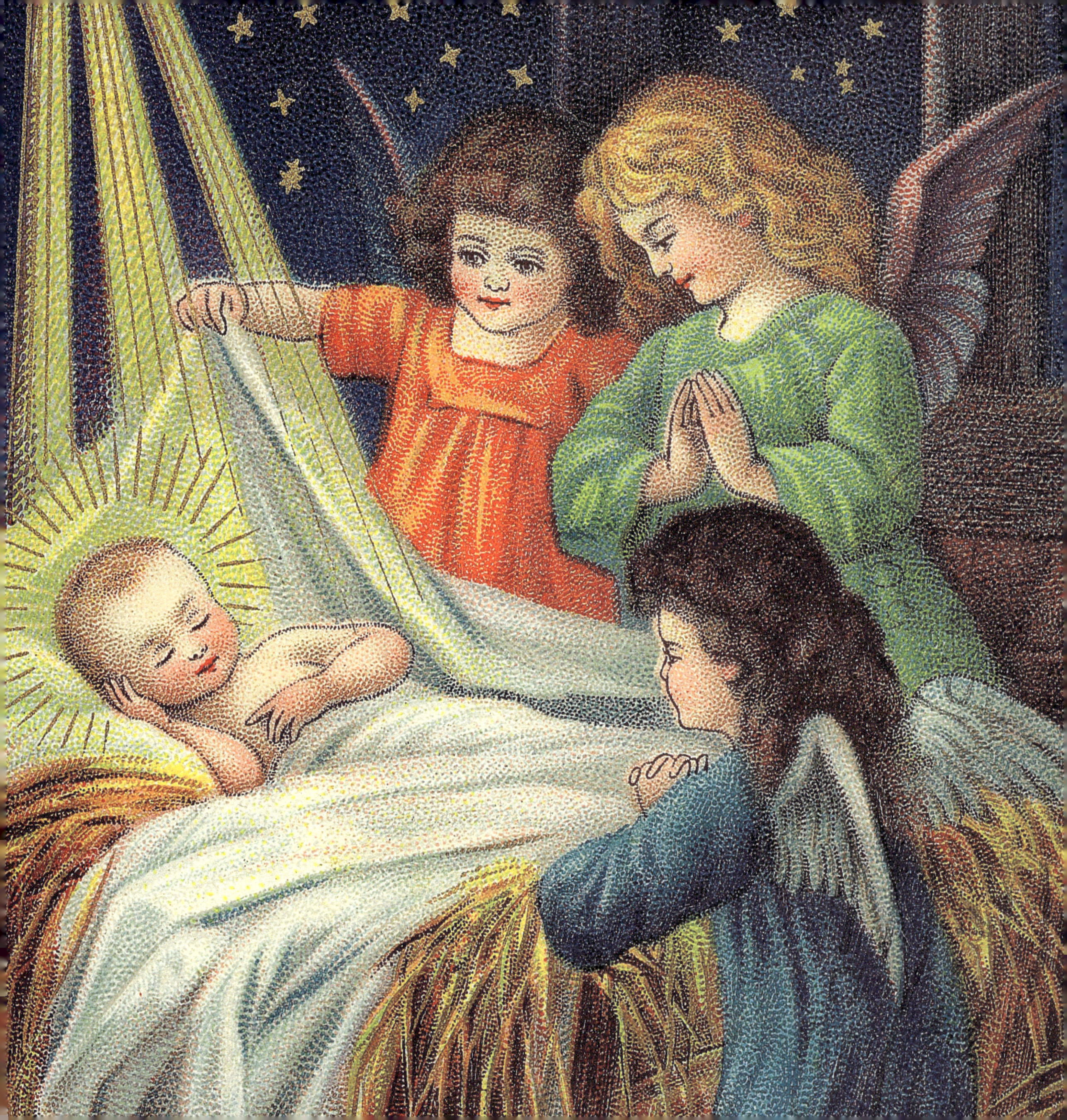

TRADITIONS: *Blessings*

Your new baby will be a blessing to you and your family. It's natural, in turn, to bless your baby at birth. In many cultures, blessings are part of a welcoming ceremony such as a bris or a baptism. Blessings also can simply be the first words that parents, family, and spiritual leaders say to newborns.

During the bris, when Jewish sons are circumcised, the father names his child and recites this blessing: "May the child [his name] grow up to Torah, to the wedding canopy and good deeds." Family and friends often express hopes that the baby was born under a good sign ("be-siman tov") or lucky star ("be-mazal tov"). Christians baptize their children to wash away "original sin" and bless them with a fresh beginning. Orthodox Christian babies are completely immersed in water three times. Roman Catholics and Anglicans anoint the baby's brow with a little water and mark a cross. In Senegal during a baby's naming ceremony, paper upon which prayers have been copied from the Koran is soaked in water. Then, before the infant is named, small pieces of the blessed paper are ripped off and placed on the baby's tongue.

The Orkney Islands offer a different take on ceremonies and blessings. After the baby is born, parents give out *blide-maet*, or "joy-food," at a feast held so friends and family can come and praise the baby and mother.

Any uttered admiration of the baby must be followed by "Guid save hid" (God save it) or "Sef bae hid" (Safe be it); otherwise, evil spirits might show unwanted attention, thinking the child too precious to live.

But a formal ceremony is not needed to bless a child. In many cultures, simple blessings are expressed by family and spiritual leaders when a baby is born. Mothers from Yemen might murmur to their infants, "My little meat, my little fat, my little honey, my grasshopper, my tiny moon, light of my eyes." Algiers midwives say, "I take the thorns from your path," three times as they pull imaginary thorns from the newborn's feet. The first words many Sikh parents utter to their babies are called the Mool Mantra:

> *There is one God, Eternal truth is his name; He made everything and is in everything. He is not afraid of anything and is not fighting anything; He is not affected by time; He was not born, He made Himself; we know about Him from the teachings of the Guru.*

A Muslim father greets his newborn by whispering the Call to Prayer, or *Adhan*, first in his child's right ear and then in the left. During birth, Navajos traditionally chant "The Blessing Way," a song meant to set the infant on a balanced, healthy, successful life path. After babies are born to Buddhist families, monks often attend the house, chanting and blessing the infant.

You will choose how you want to bless your baby. Whether it's part of a formal ceremony or just something quiet between you and your newborn, take the time to express your feelings, hopes, and prayers. And may your little blessing be forever blessed.

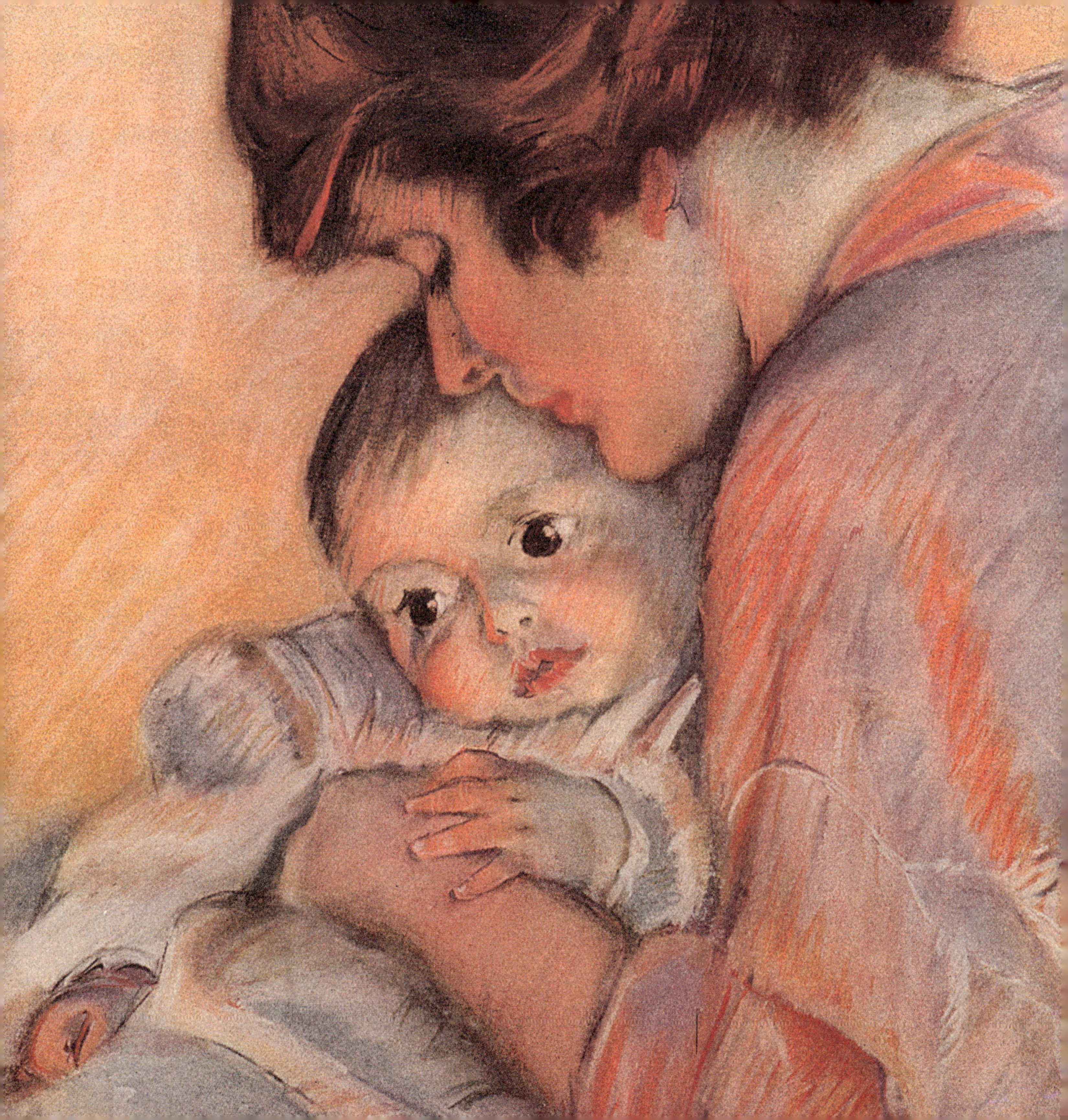

Old Wives' Tales:

Your Baby's Character

Nine months can be a long time. During this period, you'll have plenty of hours to daydream and wonder what kind of person your baby will be. Will your child be strong? Generous? Prosperous? Patient...? In case *you* are not so patient, we've polled the Old Wives and compiled some sayings that might help you influence and predict your baby's nature. Keep in mind, of course, that nature alone will have the ultimate say!

Numerous cultures believe your behavior during pregnancy can affect your child's, sex, character and physical well-being, especially when it comes to what you eat or *don't* eat. The Chinese have always believed you can influence the sex of your baby by consuming certain kinds of foods for seven days before conceiving. For a boy, dine on carrots, lettuce, mushrooms, and tofu. For a girl, eat fish, meat, and pickles. Some Native American mothers-to-be avoid berries for fear of birthmarks, steelhead salmon for fear of babies with weak ankles, and seagulls or cranes for fear of "crybabies."

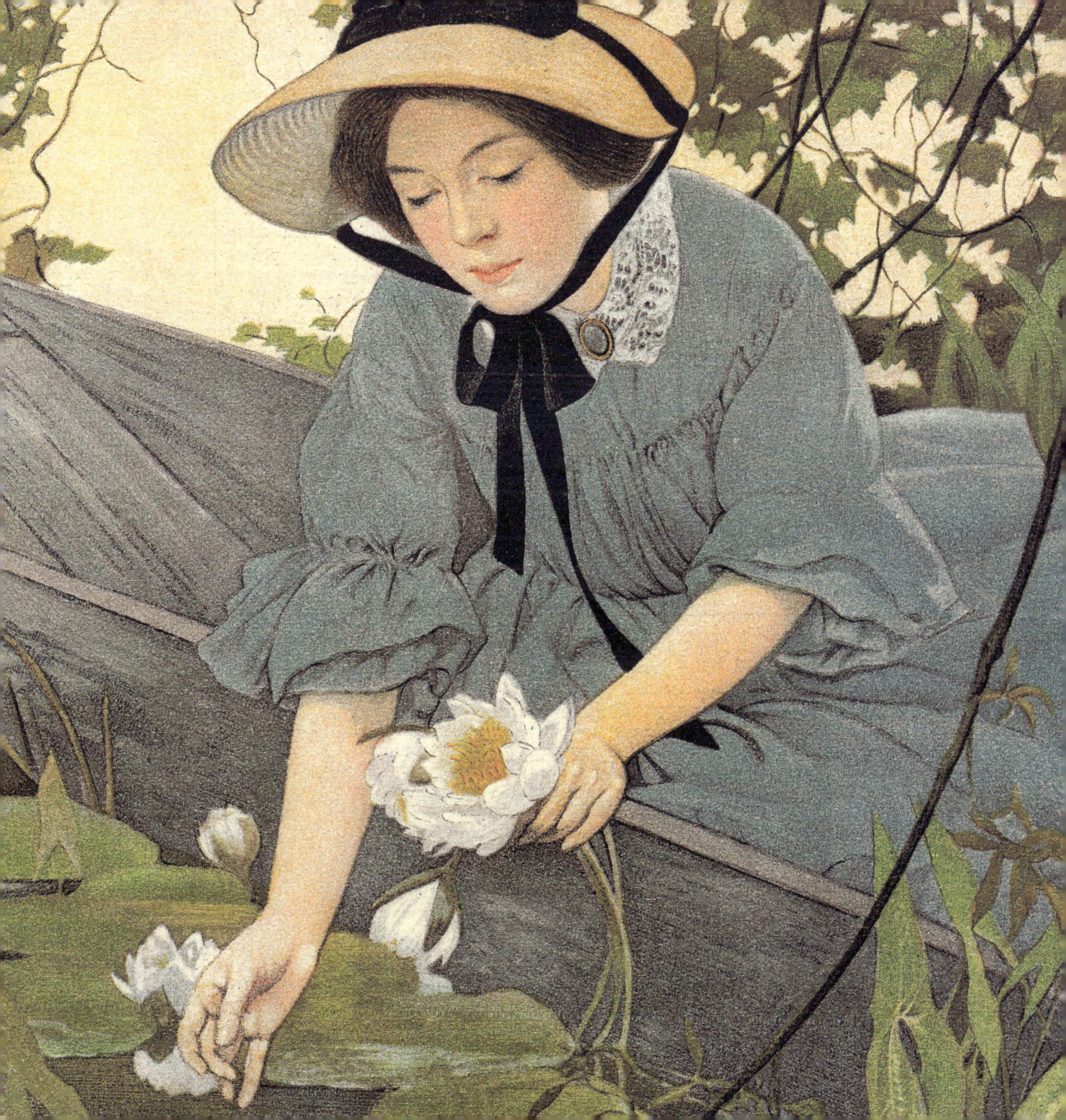

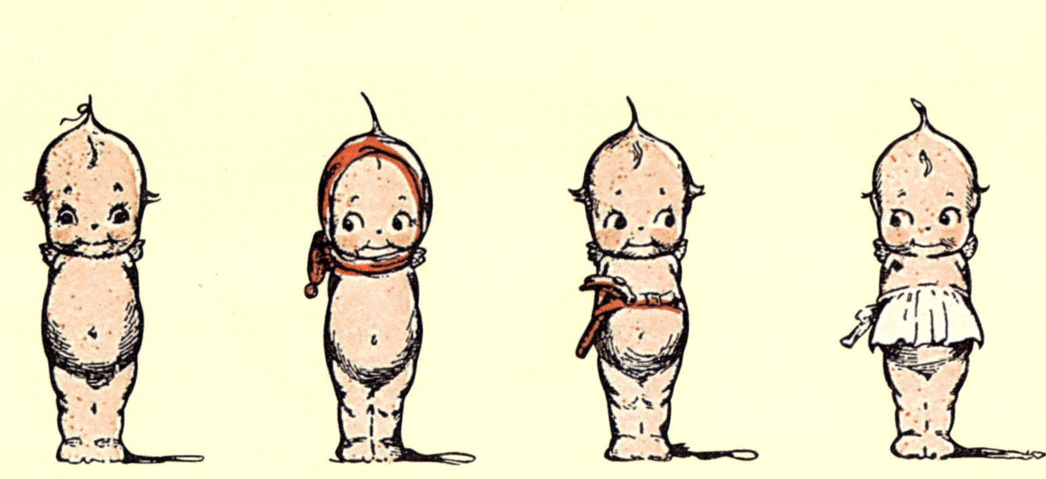

In Uganda, expectant mothers are told not to drink water while standing so their babies won't be born with squinted eyes.

If you're a believer, you'll also want to be aware of these unusual superstitions: The Aztecs believed that a pregnant woman who saw an eclipse would have a baby with a harelip; in China, a mother-to-be who rubs her belly too much might produce a spoiled, over-demanding child; and general folk wisdom asserts that happily married couples will have good-looking children, while the babies of couples who argue are fated to be less than attractive.

Some cultures say the timing of your baby's birth offers insights. In China, the hour, day, month, and year of childbirth decide which of Eight Characters the baby is born under. The Character then helps determine the baby's future success, wealth, and good fortune.

Another superstition asserts that a baby born on Sunday cannot be harmed by evil spirits. In Malta, many believe a boy born on Saint Mary's Day in August will become a great horse racer. And some say that a baby born at night will stay awake at night.

So once your baby arrives, what can you predict about personality? It is said a baby that emerges feet first will have healing abilities. A baby born

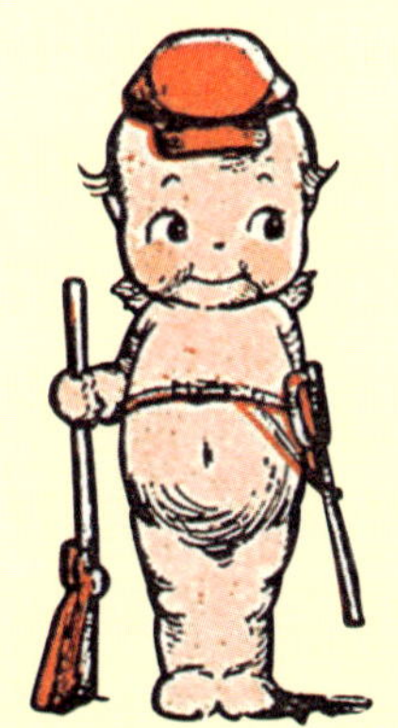
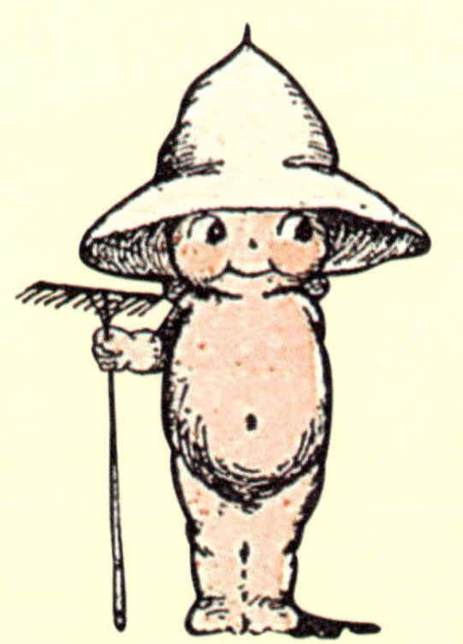
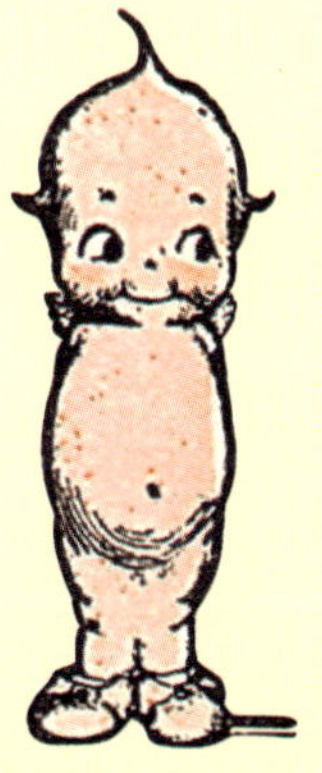
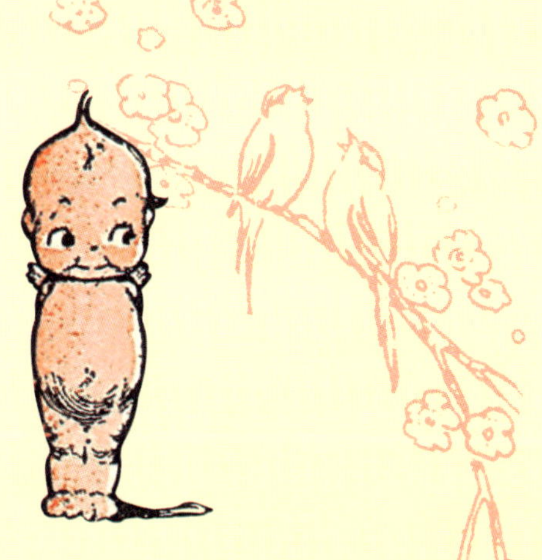

from a red water sac is believed to have great powers and double sight. Large ears foretell your baby will be generous. If your baby is born with open hands and out-stretched fingers, some see prosperity. A large mouth predicts a good singer (though beware–a baby born with teeth could grow up to be a vampire!) The Chinese say wide, thick ears or a concave navel are signs of future happiness and success. And when in doubt, parents in both China and Malta place symbolic objects like an ink well, needlework, a book, rosary beads, or an official seal in a basket and offer it to the baby. The first object the baby grabs signifies the child's destiny.

Still anxious? Well, perhaps you can influence characteristics even after your baby is born. In the Pacific's Caroline Islands, parents place the baby's umbilical cord in a conch shell they then use to influence the baby's future. For example, if parents think their child will one day need to be a good climber, they hang the conch on a tree. Germans say that a newborn laid first on her left side will grow up to be clumsy. Native American mothers were known to dunk male sons in water to assure they'd become strong, brave men and hardy hunters. And in China, rubbing a cooked chicken's tongue on your baby's lips is said to make your child a good talker.

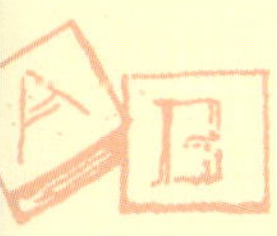
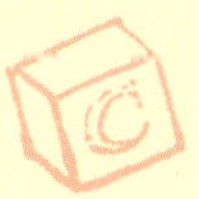

And you have dreams about your kids. You have dreams that maybe one day your kid will be up there saying, "I'd like to thank the Nobel Academy..." Then you have this other dream where your kid is going, "Ya want fries with this?"

–Robin Williams